Becoming an Aromatherapist

*The Complete Guide to training
and working in aromatherapy*

RHIANNON HARRIS
2nd edition

How To Books

Published by How To Books Ltd,
3 Newtec Place, Magdalen Road,
Oxford OX4 1RE, United Kingdom.
Tel: (01865) 793806. Fax: (01865) 248780.
email: info@howtobooks.co.uk
http://www.howtobooks.co.uk

First edition 1999
Second edition 2000

British Library Cataloguing in Publication Data.
A catalogue record for this book is available from
the British Library.

Cover design by Shireen Nathoo Design
Cover image by PhotoDisc
Cartoons by Mike Flanagan

Produced for How To Books by Deer Park Productions
Typeset by Anneset, Weston-super-Mare, N Somerset
Printed and bound by Cromwell Press, Trowbridge, Wiltshire

Contents

List of Figures and Tables

Preface

to the Second Edition

Over the past 25 years, the popularity of the aromatherapy industry has grown throughout the world and firmly established its place in the field of complementary medicine. In its wake have come numerous colleges, associations, products, suppliers, books and business opportunities. This fragrant world of aromatherapy attracts people from all walks of life. Yet for the person wanting to become an aromatherapist, very little guidance exists regarding where to start and how to take advantage of the available learning opportunities.

The aim of this updated and revised second edition is to give you encouragement, guidance, sound advice and support through all the stages of your aromatherapy experience and give you an insight of what it is like to be a therapist. The books logical, working style encourages you to participate in its content and consider issues that arise as well as stimulate thought and discussion. It is suitable for individual study or as a learning tool within a classroom setting and will continue to be of use once you are practicing aromatherapy.

This book has been written through direct experience of the various aromatherapy training opportunities that currently exist, together with the rewards and difficulties of establishing a successful career. As the aromatherapy profession continues to evolve, there will undoubtedly be changes to its various training structures and standards. This book challenges you to explore the opportunities that exist irrespective of when you enter the profession and where in the world you are based.

I trust you will find it useful reference source for many years to come.

Special thanks go to my husband, Bob, for his invaluable assistance with the illustrations and structuring of this book and the encouragement of a special friend and fellow aromatherapy educator, Lorna Dixon.

Rhiannon Harris

1

Exploring the foundations

The purpose of this initial chapter is to:

- familiarise you with different aspects of the aromatherapy profession

- introduce key subjects and concepts

- help you prepare for what lies ahead

- give you encouragement to step into a successful career.

By the end of the chapter, you will have gained a broad idea as to what the aromatherapy profession entails and will be starting to form a clear idea as to your aims and objectives in becoming an aromatherapist. The subsequent chapters will then guide you through each aspect of your training, career preparation and future prospects.

DEFINING AROMATHERAPY

Getting a grasp of the subject

The word **aromatherapy** means different things to different people. You will have already started to form your own idea as to what aromatherapy means to you. Shaped by your background, experiences and interests, this meaning has greatly influenced your decision to become an aromatherapist. It is thus helpful to examine your understanding more closely in order to evaluate how your view of aromatherapy corresponds with others in the field. In doing so, you will create a firm foundation upon which to build.

Establishing key words and concepts

The first step you need to take is to explore what aromatherapy entails. Aromatherapy has a specific language and terminology of its own.

When starting out in this rewarding therapy, it is helpful to become familiar with key words and concepts. To help get you started, Table 1 lists 36 key words related to aromatherapy commonly found in definitions around the world.

Table 1. Key words used in aromatherapy

essential oils	well-being	blending
consultation	natural	skin
massage	individual	treatment
inhalation	essence	notes
sense of smell	selection	emotional
aroma	concentrated	stress
holistic	mood	physical
pure	balance	distillation
synergy	beauty	personalised
touch	plants	health
chemistry	health	psychological
dilution	therapeutic	fragrance

Ask yourself. . .

1. Which key words match my perceptions of aromatherapy?

2. Are there key words that I would like to add to the list?

3. Are there words on this list that I do not understand?

The glossary at the end of this book explains many of these aromatherapy terms to enable you to gain a greater understanding of any key words that you do not recognise.

Making your own definition of aromatherapy

The next step is to attempt to create a definition of aromatherapy that most reflects your own experiences and expectations. The purpose of this exercise is to identify what aromatherapy means to you at the present time, rather than accept other people's opinions as your own. Identifying your starting point is always a useful reference from which to chart your progress! As you advance through your aromatherapy training and career, it will be useful to refer to and amend this initial personal definition as you develop other skills and perceptions. Using the key words you have identified above as a guide, in one or two sentences, try and **write down your own definition**. The act of writing it down will help crystallise your thoughts and create a realistic reference point.

Comparing with others

You may be surprised to learn that there is no universally accepted definition of aromatherapy. Below are some definitions from differing sources, for comparison with your own. They are not necessarily better than, or meant to replace, your definition. They merely serve as a point of discussion and stimulation of thought and further study.

● 'Aromatherapy is the use of essential oils for therapeutic purposes.' Jane Buckle, 1997.

● 'Aromatherapy is the use of essential oils to promote the health and vitality of the body, mind and spirit by inhalation, baths, compresses, topical application and massage.' Shirley Price, 1985.

● Aromatherapy may be defined as the therapeutic use of aromatic substances extracted from plants. The most important class of these substances is known as the essential oils.' Andrew Vickers, 1995.

● 'Aromatherapy is the therapeutic use of odiferous substances obtained from flowers, plants and aromatic shrubs.' Danièle Ryman, 1984.

● Aromatherapy is . . . 'the art – and science – of using plant oils in treatment.' Patricia Davis, 1995.

You will see from the above that there are two consistent themes in aromatherapy definitions:

1. essential oils
2. therapeutic effects.

Aromatherapy cannot exist without essential oils. These fragrant substances contribute to the 'aroma' part of the word. Health and/or wellbeing is always the optimal aim in their use. This forms the 'therapy' part of the word. The methods by which the essential oils are used in order to achieve health and/or well-being may vary, but the goal is always the same. This will become more apparent as the chapter progresses.

CLARIFYING THE DIFFERENT FACETS

Aromatherapy is regarded by many as an evolutionary therapy. Fragrant substances have been used around the world for their capacity to help and heal on all levels of the mind, body and spirit. With regard to aromatherapy and essential oils, depending on context and location, you will find there are different facets of this healing art.

Summarising different approaches
These different approaches are largely dependent upon the nature of the desired result, together with the background and skills of the therapist. Figure 1 demonstrates the five major facets of aromatherapy.

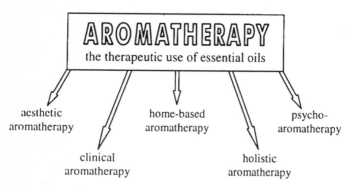

Fig. 1. The different facets of aromatherapy.

Clinical aromatherapy
Clinical aromatherapists utilise their skills within a medical environment or according to principles of orthodox medical thinking. Nurses, doctors, physiotherapists and pharmacists are examples of persons using this type of aromatherapy. A clinical aromatherapy treatment may or may not include massage to apply selected essential oils. When doctors prescribe and use essential oils in a similar way to medicines, this may be more accurately termed **medical aromatherapy** and aromatherapists who use essential oils intensively in their care are sometimes called **aromatologists**. Currently medical aromatherapy is most commonly used in France.

Holistic aromatherapy
Holistic aromatherapists tend to work within the field of alternative and complementary medicine and may have other skills such as reflexology and holistic massage. Their focus is on the promotion and maintenance of health and well-being on all levels of a person including the energetic or spiritual level. They may use philosophies of health and disease that differ from standard orthodox approaches. A typical holistic aromatherapy treatment will involve a detailed consultation with the client followed by massage to apply the selected essential oils.

Aesthetic aromatherapy
Aesthetic aromatherapists work mainly within the beauty sector and utilise essential oils to enhance their care. Essential oils have long been employed for their positive effects upon the skin. Thus the emphasis of aesthetic aromatherapy is on well-being from a predominantly beauty angle, by using essential oils in massage, skin care products and other applications.

Psycho-aromatherapy
Sometimes called **aroma chology**, this facet explores the effect of aromas on the mind and emotions, particularly via the sense of smell. This form of aromatherapy may not use massage at all. However, other approaches such as relaxation techniques and autosuggestion may be used to enhance the effects of the inhaled aromas. The effect of fragrance upon the mind and body is a subject of much interest and research, particularly in countries such as Japan and the USA.

Home-based aromatherapy
Aromatherapy is used widely by the lay person for minor health problems and general pleasure around the home. There are numerous basic books available on the subject and the current 'boom' in the concept of aromatherapy has led to an increase in products available. This is often the first 'taste' of aromatherapy that people experience. Many people enter aromatherapy training following good experiences with using essential oils at home.

From these different facets of aromatherapy, it is obvious that the level and style of training for each will be different. For example, compare the difference in skills and knowledge level necessary between a doctor prescribing essential oils and someone using essential oils to fragrance their home! These differing facets of aromatherapy are not clear-cut and separated from one another; for example, nurses frequently use holistic aromatherapy methods within their clinical practice.

Ask yourself . . .

● Which facet/s of aromatherapy am I most interested in?

Chapter 2 will help you focus on locating the training best suited to your needs, according to which aspect of this gentle art appeals to you most.

Answering common questions

Where and how do aromatherapists work?
Figure 2 briefly outlines the differing ways in which aromatherapists work. You will find further details in Chapter 6: preparing your niche. At present in the United Kingdom, most professional aromatherapists are self-employed. This situation is beginning to change as potential employers such as health authorities and leisure centres come to appreciate the advantages of having an aromatherapist as part of their team.

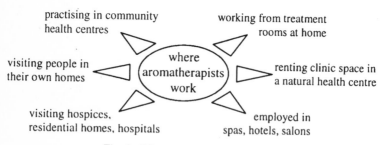

Fig. 2. Where aromatherapists work.

Who comes for aromatherapy treatments?
It is likely that your clients will be predominantly women unless you are working in a specialised environment such as a sports and fitness centre or hospital. Clients who come for aromatherapy treatments are of different ages and have a variety of needs, some of which are summarised in Figure 3.

What skills and knowledge will I need in order to practise?
This chapter briefly examines some of the qualities that an aromatherapist should strive to develop. In addition to a healthy measure of enthusiasm, commitment and drive to succeed, you will require:

AROMATHERAPY

- Specific conditions, e.g. insomnia, headaches
- General relaxation and well-being
- Pain relief
- Specific situations, e.g. bereavement, redundancy
- Recommendation from friends
- Referral from therapists or doctor
- Allied with other treatment, e.g. counselling

Fig. 3. Reasons for an aromatherapy treatment.

- knowledge of aromatherapy and essential oils

- practical skills in application of aromatherapy

- understanding of health and disease

- client handling skills

- communication skills

- business skills

- ability to liaise with other health professionals

- knowledge of matters relating to health and safety including basic First Aid

- awareness of legislation, ethics and professionalism related to therapy.

As you can see, there is much to be learnt regarding your future profession! You may already possess several of these skills; it will be up to you to adapt and develop them for the aromatherapy environment.

EXPLORING NEW CONCEPTS OF HEALTH

Introducing orthodox and unorthodox approaches
One of the requirements of an aromatherapist is that you have at least a degree of understanding of health and disease. In order to work confidently and effectively, it is important to have some awareness of how

the body works. Thus most aromatherapy courses demand that you study or have studied anatomy, physiology and pathology prior to your aromatherapy training. The level of this knowledge will be dependent upon the facet of aromatherapy you choose to study. For example, the aesthetic aromatherapist may have a different knowledge requirement of anatomy and physiology from that of an aromatologist.

Many colleges also include introductory training in different approaches to health. Called 'unorthodox' or 'alternative' therapies, these approaches may include, for example, the philosophies of Chinese and Ayurvedic medicines. Unlike orthodox medicine which is highly reliant on the physical body as being the seat of disease processes, Chinese and Ayurvedic medicines are more concerned with the restoration and maintenance of balance to the body and recognise the presence of an energetic system that influences all body processes.

Understanding holism

The words **holistic** and **holism** are frequently seen in the literature of aromatherapy and other complementary therapies. You will undoubtedly receive some form of instruction in the holistic approach during your training, irrespective of which facet you choose to study. This is because holism calls for a deep respect for the individual. It acknowledges that each person is unique and made up of many aspects that need to be nourished and kept in balance for true health to be present. Aromatherapy is thought to be useful for all these levels: physical, mental, emotional and energetic/spiritual.

Holism also recognises that each person has an innate ability to heal themselves. Aromatherapy is sometimes seen as acting as a catalyst to awaken these healing powers and thus assists the person towards balance and greater health.

Widening the parameters of health and disease

Your chosen therapy is a client-centered one. That is to say, all aspects of your client are important to you. In order to select the most appropriate essential oils for their treatment, you need to consult with them fully regarding their health, lifestyle and well-being. To illustrate this point, consider the following example:

A 'simple' matter of a headache . . .
Mrs X has come to you with recurrent headaches for which her doctor can find no organic cause. She hopes aromatherapy may be able to help.

● If you were taking a straightforward approach, that was physically-orientated rather than client-centered, you could use your reference sources to select essential oils that have pain-relieving properties after a minimum of consultation. Your treatment might be simply to massage Mrs X's head and neck with your chosen pain-relieving blend.

● Had you taken a client-centered approach, you would have discovered through consultation that Mrs X has a history of neck and shoulder stiffness for many years that seems to correlate with the severity of her headaches. Additionally, her headaches occur without fail every weekend and her job is highly stressful and unfulfilling. Your choice of essential oils may now be different from your initial selection. They would include oils that reduce spasm and stiffness as well as pain and help her deal with emotional stress. Your treatment approach may also be different. You might choose to give a deeply relaxing massage to Mrs X, whilst working on areas of her body that seem particularly tense.

By exploring all aspects of the client's health, lifestyle and circumstances, you are helping to treat the problem closer to its cause than if you had merely selected treatment for the presenting problem itself. Additionally, you are helping the client to see her problems as interrelated and thus increase her own awareness and self-responsibility.

Your aromatherapy training and experiences will undoubtedly encourage you to explore and widen your own concepts of health and disease. By retaining an open mind and remembering that the focus of treatment is client-orientated rather than disease-orientated, you will expand your potential for being a truly effective therapist.

PROFILING THE ROLE OF THE THERAPIST

Identifying key qualities

Aromatherapy is not just about essential oils and their beneficial effects. The relationship developed between the therapist and the client is an additional and essential aspect of the therapy. Thus it is worth spending a few moments examining the role of the therapist, as it is something you will develop for your future career. Table 2 lists key therapist qualities.

Table 2.   Key therapist qualities

honest	professional	knowledgeable
competent	committed	efficient
confident	non-judgmental	warm
communicative	impartial	tidy
empathetic	confidential	trustworthy
open	polite	client-centered
punctual	understanding	good listener
well groomed	adaptable	patient
friendly	consistent	reliable
prepared	organised	reassuring
welcoming	approachable	attentive
humorous	accepting	smiling
respectful	humble	unobtrusive
integrity	hygienic	calm

Ask yourself. . .

1. Out of the key qualities in Table 2, which ten qualities do I consider most important?

2. Are there any other qualities not listed that need including?

3. Can I picture myself in a therapist's role?

The qualities listed apply to a therapist of any discipline, not just aromatherapy. Therapy is by its very nature client-centered. Your client will be coming to you with particular needs that they are hoping you will meet. Thus, on some level they are vulnerable and open to negative as well as positive experiences. It is important that you ensure that your interaction with your client is of a positive nature. The client's welfare and well-being is paramount at all times.

Appreciating limitations

Having considered the qualities listed in Table 2, you may now be thinking that you will have to be all things to all people and be able to act and react appropriately in any given situation. This impression of your role is a false one and if you try to fulfil it, you are setting yourself up for disappointment. Everyone has their limitations, aromatherapists included!

It is important to work always within your sphere of competence. For example, having good listening skills and an ability to communicate as an aromatherapist does not mean you are automatically a trained counsellor and able to deal with complex emotional issues. Yet in order to know these limitations, you need first to establish clearly your levels of competence. You are a caring person by nature. Sometimes, this can lead to situations where you are tempted to take on more than you are capable of, or your client may hold you in a position of greater competence than you are able to maintain. This is a recipe for disaster! That is why it is so important to be aware of limitations and to be honest and clear about them right from the start.

In Chapter 6, you will find advice on how to establish a network with other professionals to whom you can refer your clients when you have reached the limit of your scope as an aromatherapist.

ASSESSING YOUR QUALITIES AND APTITUDES

Identifying strengths and weaknesses
Using the ten qualities you have selected from Table 2 as being the most important to you, you might like to assess your own existing qualities and aptitudes in their light. Try and place your list in the following categories:

1. qualities I already possess
2. qualities I can achieve with some effort
3. qualities that are difficult to achieve and will require much work.

At this early stage, do not expect to be able to meet each quality easily and without effort; with time, practice, commitment and awareness, you will build upon your skills. As you progress through your training and career, refer to and amend this assessment at regular intervals. The purpose is to help you in the early stages to focus your mind upon the image/role of the therapist. In doing so, you commence a period of 'grooming' for the career you intend to embrace. Aromatherapy is a voyage of self-discovery and personal development. Focusing on yourself is a useful starting point for working with others.

Using honesty in self-appraisal

Some people have a low opinion of themselves. This can lead to a distorted perception of their qualities, as they will always rate themselves lower than the true picture. If you are a highly self-critical person, ask friends and family to tell you their perceptions of your qualities. It may be that you project a very different picture than you imagine! Remember that it is the qualities that your client perceives which are particularly important.

Building on your findings

Having identified areas that you will need to develop as a therapist, the next step is to find opportunities and ways in which to do so. Your training environment should provide you with many opportunities to practise your new skills. It will be up to you to make full use of them. Take each quality in turn and ask yourself how you may develop it more fully. For example, if you have highlighted communication skills as being an area you need to develop, you may wish to:

1. talk to a counsellor in your area
2. obtain a book on communication skills from your library
3. make more time to talk with and listen to others.

SUMMARY

This chapter has been concerned with building on foundations you already possess to prepare you for the learning ahead. You will have:

- created a personal definition of what aromatherapy means to you

- looked at different aspects of aromatherapy and how it is practised

- gained an insight into differing approaches to health

- considered the role of the therapist

- gained some awareness of the client-centered approach at the heart of the therapy

- assessed some of your existing therapist qualities and aptitudes.

CASE STUDIES

Jane looks for a career change

Jane is 26 years old, single and currently unemployed. She is looking for a total career change following redundancy. She describes her previous job as a bank clerk as 'impersonal' and 'unfulfilling' and is looking to develop her interest in complementary therapies. She has received differing treatments over the years for a number of problems and found aromatherapy particularly beneficial for stress relief. She is looking forward to a new career that involves a person-centered approach.

Theresa chooses to regain some independence

Theresa is 46 years old, married and has two children in college. She lives in a detached house in the country. She is interested in learning more about aromatherapy with a view to being able to treat family and friends and possibly earn 'a bit of pocket money'. She has considerable free time on her hands and is anticipating the time when her children leave home.

Mark is looking to extend his skills

Mark is 22 years old, single and a qualified sports therapist, masseur and gym instructor. He currently works full-time at a local leisure centre and has heard that aromatherapy may help his clients. He has never had an aromatherapy treatment himself although his partner and several clients have told him of its efficacy. He is interested in undertaking a course in order to integrate new skills to enhance his work.

THINKING IT THROUGH

1. Take the time to write a short paragraph about why you want to be an aromatherapist and what aspect of this therapy you are particularly interested in.

2. Suggest three ways in which you can develop each of your therapist qualities.

3. Having now worked through this introductory chapter, consider whether the overview meets with your initial preconceptions about what is involved in an aromatherapy career.

2

Getting Started

This chapter is concerned with helping you make the right choice of course and getting you started on the road to a successful career. Chapter 1 helped you consider which facet of the therapy most appeals to you and gave you an overview of what the aromatherapy profession involves. It is now time to move on and consider how to locate the most appropriate training for your needs. In order to locate something, though, you first need to know clearly what you are looking for!

ASSESSING YOUR MOTIVES

Examining your reasons

One of the first questions to ask yourself is why you want to be an aromatherapist. By identifying precisely your needs and expectations, you will be in a better position to find the right training. Many people enter the therapy profession without a clear idea as to what they want out of their course and career and subsequently end up being disappointed or paying for something they are not suited for. Thus it is time to be completely honest with yourself. There are four main categories regarding a person's decision to enter a therapy career:

1. social

2. financial

3. personal

4. professional.

No one category is entirely separate from the other; often a person chooses to train as an aromatherapist for several of the reasons outlined above. However, it is likely that one reason outweighs the others, thus giving you an idea of the balance of your motives. Look at the various factors behind each category in Table 3 and then ask yourself which motives most apply to you.

Table 3. Motives for becoming an aromatherapist

Social	Financial
to acquire skills in stress management	to earn a part-time or full-time income
to educate others regarding a holistic lifestyle	to develop a product line
to develop meaningful communication skills	to sell essential oils
to empower people	to increase product knowledge
to broaden experience of a natural therapy	to follow popular opinion and interests
to gain more meaningful contact with people	to write articles or books on the subject
to help those in need, e.g. elderly, cancer care	to become an aromatherapy teacher
to give back something to society	to increase job prospects
Personal	**Professional**
to expand an existing interest	to offer aromatherapy in the workplace
to improve self-esteem	to extend the role as a therapist/nurse/healer
to gain respect and recognition	to develop specialist skills, e.g. pain control
to further personal development	to continue professional development
to improve personal health	to increase my product knowledge
to make more friends and contacts	to augment my existing skills
to extend existing skills and qualifications	to learn a new skill

Weighing up

Using Table 3, are your reasons for becoming an aromatherapist more in one category than another? It may help to circle, underline or add to the reasons to assist with defining your motives.

If your reasons are predominantly social

You may require a course with a largely client-centered approach with great emphasis on communication skills such as counselling, massage and healing. You may wish to explore the potentials of other complementary therapies and study subjects such as nutrition and stress management. The size of class may be important to you; large enough to allow expression and interchange of ideas yet small enough to encourage and foster a group identity. It is unlikely that a distance-learning aromatherapy course will meet your social needs. Your chosen course may become an open door, leading you into study of other subjects. It may be that the time-frame for completion is not particularly important – part-time or extended courses are often most suitable for socially orientated students.

If your reasons are predominantly financial

You may wish to choose a course with more clearly defined objectives and one that offers in depth support and training in business skills, marketing and promotion. You need to be sure that the course equips you with as many skills as possible to survive financially. The time frame for completion will also be important; condensed, full-time courses are popular with those looking for a career in aromatherapy. The qualification you receive will be important to ensure that it is recognised by members of the public and the profession in general. You will need to choose a course that has been accredited by an aromatherapy association.

If your reasons are predominantly personal

You may wish to choose a course with a highly experiential content that has a student support group. Its emphasis will be to encourage you to explore your own patterns and balance on all levels and develop a personalised approach to using essential oils and aromatherapy. The course may involve other subjects such as healing, body massage, counselling and holistic approaches to health. The course may be lengthy, and lead you on to other aspects of health care. A distance-learning course may be a suitable choice, enabling you to progress at your own pace with full support from the tutors and other students who may be at different stages from you and in different parts of the world.

If your motives are purely professional
It is likely that you are looking for a specific type of aromatherapy training. This may include a clinical aromatherapy course if you are a nurse
or an essential oils course if you are a beautician, essential oil retailer or
herbalist. The time-scale for completion is likely to be relatively short,
leading to a certificate of attendance or full qualification. You may
already have skills and training that will be recognised and lead to
exemptions from parts of the course you choose to undertake.

MAKING THE CHOICE OF COURSE

Knowing your options
There are two main options when considering entering aromatherapy
training in the UK: you can embark on a course of study with either a
private or a non-private aromatherapy college. Both have relative advantages and disadvantages as can be seen in Table 4.

Concerning national standards
In the UK there are now national occupational standards developed
specifically for aromatherapy practitioners, although they have yet to be
implemented. You may thus find several colleges are already paving the
way for incorporating these standards into their training, leading to
National Vocational Qualifications at level three. This may or may not
influence your choice of course. A copy of the national occupational
standards for aromatherapy can be obtained from the Local Government
Management Board. See the Useful Addresses and Resource Guide for
further details.

LOCATING THE BEST TRAINING FOR YOUR NEEDS

Using your resources
There are many ways to find out about aromatherapy courses in your
area. Consider the following list of resources:

- local library
- centres of adult education
- health magazines
- professional journals, e.g. aromatherapy, nursing, beauty
- local aromatherapists

Table 4. Advantages and disadvantages of aromatherapy training establishments

PRIVATE EDUCATION
Advantages C
Independent college — varied courses
Personal tuition a possibility
Part-time or full-time choice
Possibility of distance learning
May specialise in the subject
Purpose-equipped premises
Flexible training programme
Possible postgraduate support

Disadvantages ☹
More expensive than non-private
Variable quality courses on offer
Not regulated or externally assessed

NON-PRIVATE EDUCATION
Advantages ☺
Local college/university
NVQ-style training likely
Part-time and evening class
Training level recognised by other colleges
Set syllabus and curriculum
Access to other facilities on campus
Good student support
Cheaper courses

Disadvantages ☹
Facilities may not be purpose-equipped
Overall standard may be lower
Unlikely to have full-time training available
Unlikely to provide postgraduate support

- friends

- aromatherapy associations

- natural health exhibitions

- health food stores

- local special interest groups

- books on aromatherapy and natural health care

- *Yellow Pages*

- Internet sources.

You will find further details in the Useful Addresses and Resource Guide at the back of the book. Once you have obtained names and addresses, it is time to start looking more closely to find a course that meets your particular requirements.

Refining your choice

By this stage, you should have a reasonable idea as to the type of training you are looking for. Now is the time to match the course with these requirements. Most colleges, if you telephone them, will send you a course prospectus or details. This is a good way to begin refining your choice. In addition to your identified needs, you may wish to consider the following points once you receive the course details.

Getting to know the college

How promptly and efficiently a college deals with your request for information may be a useful indicator, together with the presentation of the information that is sent to you. You should expect a professional response from a professional training establishment. You may also be influenced in your choice by the reputation and standing of the college, the calibre and experience of its tutors and the length of time the course has been running. Additional information about the college that may be helpful is whether they have selection criteria or offer other courses that may be more suitable for you.

Learning more about the course

Important details such as course content, structure and length should be readily available in the prospectus, together with dates for the next available training. You need to have an idea as to the number of in-class hours taught as well as anticipated hours for home study. The approximate number of students in each class may vary; some aromatherapy associations stipulate a maximum class size to ensure adequate supervision for practical skills. Facilities to aid learning should also be listed such as the presence of a library or access to computers. Additionally, ask what your training will lead to in terms of qualification and registration.

Getting there

Another detail worth exploring is the travelling involved to attend classes. You will need to find out about possible routes using public and private transport, together with parking availability and related costs.

Asking about finances

Details regarding the costs of the course are usually included with the prospectus. Bear in mind that there are likely to be 'hidden extras' in the form of books, uniforms and compulsory course materials. You will also have to consider costs of travel and food/refreshments during class times. Chapter 3 gives you further advice on financial matters.

Ascertaining the outcome

Information regarding your future qualification should be readily provided, together with details of examinations and registration with aromatherapy or other associations as appropriate. You need to know what sort of skills the course is designed to equip you with.

Taking the plunge

Having now selected a few colleges or training centres that appear most to fulfil your needs, it is highly recommended that you arrange an informal visit of the site. Usually, this is done by telephone followed by a written confirmation as to time and location. If you are unsure where the college is, ask for both verbal and written directions. It is particularly helpful to ask if it is possible to visit when there is a class in session; this will allow you to gain an idea of class size and a clear image of the role you will have as a student.

Ask if you can meet the principal tutor of your proposed course. If you are a person with special needs such as wheelchair access or adaptations for the hard of hearing, it is particularly important to discuss these requirements with the college principal.

While you are at the site, take the fullest opportunity to gather as much information as you can. Prepare questions in advance that will help you ascertain whether the course or college meets your identified needs.

The college, in return, should be able to readily provide you with further information to help you make your choice.

Applying for the course

Having visited the college and allowed time for reflection, the next step is to confirm your application for the course. Usually, this is done in writing and may involve completing preprepared forms and paying a non-refundable deposit with the application. Most colleges prefer your application to be made in your own handwriting as opposed to typed. If so, ensure it is legible! You may be asked to write a brief summary of why you want to be an aromatherapist and how you plan to use your skills. The suggested exercise at the start of this chapter will be helpful in identifying your motives and goals.

Recognising existing skills

As there are several components to an aromatherapy training that are shared by other courses in health care, you may have already received training in a subject for which you may be exempt in your aromatherapy course. This will save you both time and money and places value on your previous knowledge and experience. Subjects common to several therapies include:

- counselling skills
- First Aid
- nursing or other training in anatomy, physiology and pathology
- nutrition
- massage.

If you already hold qualifications or have studied any of these subjects and wish to apply for exemption, you will have to demonstrate evidence of your prior training such as copies of work, certificates from other courses and other documentation. The college may also require you to take a written or practical test to confirm that you are eligible for exemption.

ANSWERING IMPORTANT QUESTIONS

Is a career in aromatherapy guaranteed to be successful?

This depends upon your definition of success! It also depends upon how much commitment, stamina and sticking power you have, in addition to your skills as a therapist. What is guaranteed is that you have entered a rewarding profession where you will learn much about yourself and others. In realistic financial terms, expect to create a stable clientele over a period of one to two years. It is rare for the new aromatherapist to find instant financial success. With the popularity of aromatherapy and the level of public awareness you will not have a shortage of clients in the long-term if you find your niche and are able to promote your skills. Careful financial planning and practice management are essential.

Will my training be recognised worldwide?

As aromatherapy is largely an unregulated profession, at present, there is no worldwide governing body for aromatherapy and thus no worldwide-accepted standards. If you intend to study in one country and utilise your skills in another, it is wise first to confirm that your qualifications will be recognised within the area in which you intend to work. For example, those who qualify as aromatherapists in the UK may have difficulty obtaining licences to practise in certain states of America. If you live outside the UK, find out if your country has an aromatherapy association and gain advice as to training standards required for you to practise. If there is no such association, you will need to make inquiries at local or county government level. The Useful Addresses and Resource Guide gives details of various aromatherapy associations around the world.

Is a diploma better than a certificate?

You will find a whole range of attractive awards, titles and designations on offer by different aromatherapy colleges. They all serve to influence and attract prospective students and may imply by their name that they are better or more accepted than other courses available. In reality, there is little or no difference between a diploma or a certificate. All they mean is that you have met the educational requirements in order to complete the course successfully. Of course, these standards are variable and educational requirements will vary from course to course; some will be harder to attain than others. What is *more* important is the quality of the course that you undertake and what recognition you receive at the end of it, not the name or elaborate design of the certificate or diploma.

SUMMARY

Choosing and locating the right aromatherapy course takes time and care. This chapter has helped you consider:

● your motives

● your needs

● your options

● the resources available

● the basic steps to selection and enrolment.

Chapter 3 is concerned with the financial aspects of your course, career and future prospects.

CASE STUDIES

Jane quickly identifies her needs

Jane is clear that she needs a top quality aromatherapy qualification that will permit her to be registered with an aromatherapy association. As she wants to make aromatherapy her career, she is looking for a full-time course that includes business skills and is prepared to travel outside her local area to study. She starts making lists of colleges from a popular health magazine and contacts her national aromatherapy associations for lists of registered colleges. Having made a short list from looking at prospectuses, she is now writing off to three colleges for an informal visit and interview.

Theresa targets her local area

For Theresa, the reasons for becoming an aromatherapist are predominantly social and personal. She is thus looking to find a course that will allow her to progress at her own pace and explore different aspects of healthcare and healing. She does not wish to have to travel far for the course. Upon speaking to her own aromatherapist and visiting her local library, she discovers a local private college that has a flexible, modular approach to aromatherapy training. She telephones the college principal to arrange a visit.

Mark looks for recognition of prior learning

Mark's reasons for studying are purely professional; he wishes to incorporate the use of essential oils within his existing practice. He is looking for a college that will recognise his existing skills and qualifications in anatomy, physiology, sports therapy and body massage. Additionally, he requires a course that will fit in with his already busy schedule. He becomes interested in an aromatherapy course conducted by evening classes that is advertised at the leisure centre where he works. He arranges a meeting with the tutor.

THINKING IT THROUGH

1. Jane, Theresa and Mark have each made an arrangement to visit and meet the course tutors before making a final decision. Why do you think this may be important?

2. Compile your own checklist and questions ready for visiting your selected colleges.

3. In the case of colleges offering courses by distance learning, it is unlikely that you will be able to visit or interview the staff directly. What other factors might influence your decision making process in this situation?

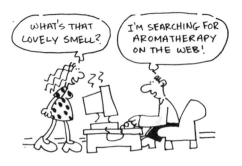

3

Counting the Cost

You may be surprised to find a chapter on business so early on in your steps to becoming an aromatherapist. Many people start off full of enthusiasm for their chosen path without considering if it is a viable option in either the short or long term. One key to success is **to be prepared on all levels**. It is particularly pertinent for the therapist to deal with issues of finances from the very outset, as this is an area that many find most difficult and challenging. This chapter will help you plan constructively and build confidence and positive thinking into your financial life.

BECOMING BUSINESS MINDED

One of the most common reasons why aromatherapists-to-be do not complete their training or fail to launch a successful career is a lack of business sense and planning. The therapy draws people from all walks of life and of varying business experience. Not all people are naturally business minded, but it is possible for everyone to develop some skills in this area. Some, but not all, colleges of aromatherapy provide adequate advice and training on this essential aspect of therapy. Often this advice comes too late; the time when you will need the most business advice and make the biggest financial outlay is in order to pay for your chosen course! Additionally, many people have unresolved fears and anxieties surrounding money and financial success. This inevitably impinges on their self-esteem and future potential.

Being your own business manager

Part of the role of an aromatherapist is to be accountable for all your actions. This is a particularly apt statement when considering finances! This is a skill that you will acquire, providing you give it time, attention and commitment. Being your own business manager will help you work more efficiently, instil confidence and give you a clear projection for your future career.

In Chapters 1 and 2, you questioned your qualities, aptitude and motives for becoming an aromatherapist. Thus you have already taken the first steps to being your own business manager. You have established an idea as to what you hope to gain from your chosen profession. Your motives may not be entirely financially driven; nevertheless a degree of financial control is still necessary. The following case examples illustrate how even those with seemingly non-financial ideals require a degree of business sense.

A case of two aromatherapists...

Aromatherapist A is a caring and well-qualified therapist. She entered the profession to 'give back' some love and care to the world and wishes to do so by offering her services on a voluntary basis. She approaches a local hospice and offers her time and expertise to the clients and their families. She proposes to provide her time, essential oils and equipment, towels and her own transport for half a day, twice weekly. The hospice manager readily accepts the offer.

Aromatherapist B is a caring and well-qualified therapist. She entered the profession to 'give back' some love and care to the world and wishes to do so by offering her services on a voluntary basis. She approaches several hospices and offers her time and expertise on a regular basis for a six-month trial period to the clients and their families. She is prepared to donate her time and expertise but requires help with the additional costs such as laundry expenses, essential oils and travel. One of the hospices agrees to buy a stock of essential oils for hospice use, provide linen and laundry facilities and pay her petrol expenses based upon mileage used.

Having read through the above real-life scenarios, ask yourself. . .

1. Which therapist is most likely to be able to 'give' the most in the long term?

2. Which therapist is most likely to be valued or undervalued?

3. Which therapist is truly in control?

To find out, let us return to follow their progress six months later . . .

Aromatherapist A started well and enthusiastically. She quickly developed a therapeutic relationship with the hospice clients and their families. Working with the sick and their carers is a very demanding but rewarding experience and she found she was giving more time than originally planned. Initially, she did not mind and stayed on long after her agreed hours. She discovered that her clients regularly needed the most expensive essential oils such as rose, neroli and frankincense. Initially, she willingly used them, despite the expense to herself. The hospice manager, pleased with the satisfaction expressed by the clients, suggested she might also like to work at the sister hospice in a neighbouring area. *Aromatherapist A* found it hard to refuse and was ashamed to mention that her finances and time were starting to become severely restricted. After six months, she was drained physically, emotionally, energetically and financially. Tired, resentful and disappointed in herself, she left the profession, berating herself for not being 'more caring' and wondering what went wrong.

Aromatherapist B started well and enthusiastically. She quickly developed a therapeutic relationship with the hospice clients and their families. She helped to establish an aromatherapy fund to help pay for the oils used in the hospice and to cover her other costs such as travel. Freed from this burden, she was able to truly 'give' of her time and expertise to those who needed it. As her role was clearly established, she worked more efficiently and her treatment hours were adhered to. She negotiated a special discount with her essential oil supplier to provide the hospice with the essential oils needed. This included the costly, precious essential oils so much required in a hospice environment. After her six months trial period ended, the hospice invited her to become part of their team – employed part-time as the hospice aromatherapist. They also invited her to act as aromatherapy co-ordinator for other hospices in the area.

Both of these aromatherapists may have received the same level of training and been motivated by the same goals and desires, but their outcomes are truly different. Why do you think this is?

- Aromatherapist B was **business minded**. She recognised that in order to truly give of herself, she also needed to receive. In her case, she was able to plan ahead and work out the realistic cost of 'giving' her time and expertise to the hospice. In doing so, she was able to put together a proposal that ultimately led to long-term benefits for all involved.

- Aromatherapist A was not business minded. Despite being a talented therapist, she did not consider the true cost of her giving in realistic financial terms. She found herself over-stretched on all levels and unable to work to her fullest potential as a result of lack of planning and assertion. In the short term, she was able to bring benefits but this could not be sustained into the long term.

The above scenarios may have helped you to recognise the need to be business minded. It is possible to retain your caring approach whilst realistically counting the cost.

Developing a business sense

You are about to spend considerable time and money embarking upon a period of training that will lead to your goal. Once you are a qualified aromatherapist, you will need to value your skills and experience sufficiently to make a successful career. You will require enthusiasm, commitment, expertise and a business sense to succeed. Wealth does not have to be your main goal and certainly does not guarantee you happiness and security. Yet it is essential that you develop a healthy attitude towards money. Many therapists have deep-seated negative attitudes towards money and this, coupled with a low self-esteem, is a surefire way to ensure you never earn enough to maintain your career and give you the freedom to grow professionally.

Do you have a negative view about money? Consider the common belief statements in Figure 4.

Ask yourself. . .

1. Which of the statements in Figure 4 do I most identify with?
2. Are there other statements that I would like to add?

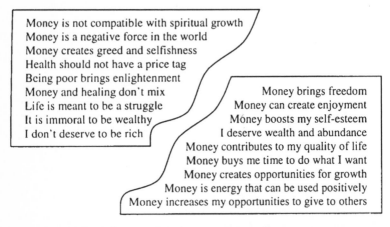

Money is not compatible with spiritual growth
Money is a negative force in the world
Money creates greed and selfishness
Health should not have a price tag
Being poor brings enlightenment
Money and healing don't mix
Life is meant to be a struggle
It is immoral to be wealthy
I don't deserve to be rich

Money brings freedom
Money can create enjoyment
Money boosts my self-esteem
I deserve wealth and abundance
Money contributes to my quality of life
Money buys me time to do what I want
Money creates opportunities for growth
Money is energy that can be used positively
Money increases my opportunities to give to others

Fig. 4 Common belief statements regarding money.

3. Do they tell me that I need to further refine my business sense and develop a more healthy approach to money?

Keeping track of finances

A wise move right from the beginning is to keep a regular record of everything financial, whether it is flowing into or out of your account. To begin with, a simple IN and OUT book may be all that is required. On the left-hand page, list all the money you receive (income). On the right-hand page, list all the money you spend (expenditure). As time goes on, you can further refine your bookkeeping skills with the help of an accountant. With all account keeping, the key phrase is to '**keep receipts for everything**'.

This is a good start to practice management. Providing you keep accurate records and receipts, there are many things you can claim against tax as business expenses. These include:

● All running costs of your business such as heating, lighting, telephone bill, advertising, and rent of premises. Costs of upkeep and maintenance of business premises are also included such as basic decorating and repairs.

● All business stationery, postage, promotional literature, books, journal subscriptions, membership fees, conference and seminar costs.

● Transport costs, particularly if you are a mobile therapist where your car is an essential part of your business. You may be able to claim a percentage of repair work and car tax as well as fuel bills. If you travel to seminars or conferences, you may also claim your travel expenses to and from the event.

● Certain forms of entertainment may also be claimed on the business, such as your overnight stay prior to a conference, plus breakfast and dinner. A limited amount is also allowed for gifts and staff entertainment per year.

● All equipment required for the running of the business such as essential oils and related products, massage couch, linen, protective clothing/uniform and sundries such as soap and toilet paper.

● Professional fees such as those paid to your accountant or solicitor, and bank charges on your business account. You may also claim the costs of insurance for yourself and your premises with regard to your work.

As you can see, there are good reasons for keeping those receipts! Your accountant will be able to further advise you on other expenses that are permissible on the business. These will all go forward to being offset against tax, thus saving you money.

Another wise move is to open a bank account to be used solely for your aromatherapy course and career. This will help later when it comes to accounting and keeps a clear distinction between your business affairs and your personal life.

Finding an accountant

Many successful therapists use the services of an accountant and/or a financial adviser. He or she will be able to advise you on taxation matters and give guidance on keeping clear and accurate accounts. The accountant will also help you save money by telling you what you can legally offset against tax.

Of course, for this service, you will be charged a fee. If you are able to complete normal monthly accounts yourself, these fees will be considerably reduced. Finding a good accountant whom you can trust and who is able to meet your small business needs is important. Ask around your family and friends to see if they know of one they can recommend. Alternatively, your local library or bank manager will be able to provide details of accountants and financial advisers in your area.

Balancing the equation

The art of business is to ensure that, at the very least, your income exceeds your expenditure! You must be prepared to be patient for this to happen and to work actively towards this goal. In the initial stages, as with most small businesses, there will be a period when your expenditure exceeds your income. The aromatherapy profession is no exception to the rule. It takes an average of two years to build a successful practice and career. This is why realism, careful business planning and budgeting are necessary right from the very beginning. For this reason, many therapists continue with part-time jobs whilst they are studying and during the initial stages of their career.

BUDGETING FOR YOUR NEW VENTURE

In an ideal world, we should not have to concern ourselves with bank balances, accounts, fees and paying taxes. However, by now you will appreciate that this is part and parcel of the life of the therapist.

Although possibly the least enjoyable aspect of your chosen therapy, it is essential. You have two choices; hate it or learn to like it!

Estimating the cost

The best place to start considering finances and gaining a business-like attitude towards your goal is right at the beginning when considering embarking on your career as an aromatherapist. Here is a practical suggestion to get you started. . .

With pen, paper and calculator, make a note of all possible expenses you will incur in order to start your aromatherapy training. Try not to miss anything out. Watch out for those 'hidden extras' that may significantly increase your expenditure. Table 5 can be used as a guide to calculating possible costs but will need to be modified or extended to meet your individual needs. The table lists 2000 prices to give a comparison but is not a substitute for your own individual costing.

Planning ahead

The next step is to extend this list to include expenses that will be incurred when you qualify and launch your career. There are no short-cuts or easy steps to this process, but in doing so, you are well on

Table 5. Estimating the cost of your course

Subject	Average cost (£)	Your cost
Course fee	500 to 2500	
Additional books	50 to 125	
Uniform	25 to 50	
Essential oil kit	115 to 200	
Massage couch	200 to 400	
Linen and sundries	30 to 60	
Student insurance	30 to 40	
Examination fees	50 per subject	
Student memberships		
Travel costs	variable	
Additional costs		

your way to creating an accurate and realistic business plan and working out how much to charge for your treatments. Here is a list of additional expenses that you may incur with qualifications.

- membership of professional bodies
- subscription to professional magazines
- loan repayments
- insurance
- accountants fees
- National Insurance contributions if you are self-employed in the UK
- laundry
- travel
- rent of premises
- stationery and promotional literature
- advertising
- licence to practise fees (check with your local council)
- essential oils and related products
- bottles, jars and blending equipment.

The above list is purely for reference to get you started; it is suggested you make your own personalised list. The more thorough you are, the more accurate your plan will be.

Making a business plan

A business plan enables you to put all the information you have just gathered into a projection and proposal for your future career. Creating a business plan may seem a daunting prospect at first but it will prove an invaluable tool. A business plan has three main purposes:

1. It brings into focus your realistic needs and goals and gives you a blueprint to work from.

2. It is useful to refer to periodically to assess whether you are achieving your aims.

3. It is necessary if you require financial assistance to fund your course and future plans.

The formats for business plans vary in style and length but the essential information remains the same. Business plan outlines accompany most small business information packs that are freely available from banks and small business advice centres. You may wish to collect a few such plans to familiarise yourself with their format and level of detail required. Alternatively, you may create your own. Detailed below is the basic information required in every business plan.

Information about yourself
This is the 'who' part of the business plan. It should reflect your background, personal ambitions, commitments, reputation and the reasons why you have chosen to become an aromatherapist. Business plans are not just about money. Your bank manager or sponsor will want to have confidence in you, your abilities and your professionalism. Your personal assessments conducted in Chapters 1 and 2 will help you clearly establish your strengths and motives.

Information about your business
This is where the detailed information you have been gathering is important. This is the 'what, why, when, where and how'of the business plan! You will need to explain clearly:

● What is the nature and objective of your business, and the market that exists for your skills.

● Why you feel you can achieve success in this area.

● When you plan to commence business/training.

● Where you intend to operate, including details of premises, equipment needed, together with costings.

● How you plan to operate. This will include cash flow forecasts (what you foresee flowing into and out of your account) for approximately two years and a full breakdown of costs.

● Information about your future plans. In business, your eyes need to be trained on the horizon as well as on the realities of everyday life. You will need to include information on how you see your business evolving and expanding.

Your financial requirements

You need to state clearly how much money you require for the initial outlay and your working capital. You also need to state how you intend to fund and repay it. These details will be based upon all the information you have already put into the business plan. Do not be tempted to under-price your needs. Unrealistic or inaccurate costing may ultimately put you out of business.

Seeking independent business advice

- **The Small Business Adviser** in your bank will be able to advise you on most financial issues.

- **The Department of Trade and Industry** provide a range of free publications covering all aspects of the subject, designed to help you develop a greater business sense. They also operate a Small Firms Loan Guarantee Scheme and have set up local Business Links to provide reliable advice from independent Personal Business Advisers.

- **The Small Business Bureau** is a lobby organisation in the UK that offers a range of services to its members. They are particularly keen to encourage the further development of women starting up in business and publish advice and articles in their *Small Business Newspaper*.

ASSESSING YOUR WORTH

One of the more difficult aspects of your business affairs is deciding how much your service is worth. Bear in mind that once you have decided upon a fee to charge, it will be difficult to change. Thus your fee needs to be realistic right from the start.

Valuing yourself

As discussed, many people have complicated attitudes towards money and their own self-worth. If you are someone who feels uncomfortable about charging for your treatments, it is particularly important for you to develop a way of coping with this. You need to separate your emotions from the act of taking money for your services. Remember that if you under-price your work, you will undermine your abilities.

Do not think that by charging less for your treatment, you will attract more clients. It usually works in reverse! If you are 'cheaper' than the other therapists in your locality, it may be perceived that the treatment you offer is of inferior quality. Your charges need to reflect the commitment you have made to studying, setting up in practice and your professional attitude towards your work.

Comparing prices

One essential aspect of assessment is comparison with others. Conduct some market research in the locality where you intend to practise. You will find further advice regarding this in Chapter 6. Find out other practitioners' charges and what services they offer. Take into account the length of the treatments that they give and where they operate from, and try to gain some idea of their overheads. For example, one therapist who charges less may be operating from their home, in contrast to a therapist operating from a clinic whose prices will reflect the greater costs of running her practice. Gain as much information as you can, as this will help you in the next step: charging the right amount.

Charging the right amount

Figure 5 gives you some idea of the factors you will need to take into account when working out how much to charge. It is not an easy task, but is essential if you are going to make a living out of working as an aromatherapist.

PAYING FOR YOUR COURSE

Choosing the best means of payment

Having gained a clearer picture of your financial future, it is necessary to consider how to pay for your course. You may be in the position of having sufficient savings to invest in your new career. If so, treat it as a loan from yourself to your business that will need to be repaid. In this way, you maintain a business-like approach to your new career.

You may not be in the position of being able to fund the course and launch your career single-handed. Instead, you require financial assistance from an outside source. This is a common situation for many therapists; a realistic business plan will be essential to help you determine precisely how much you need to borrow and the sensible repayment period you will require.

There are a number of options and schemes for borrowing money and it will be necessary to explore which one is most suitable for you.

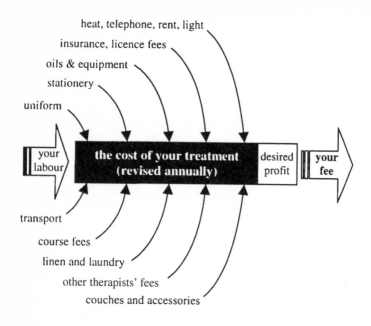

Fig. 5. Calculating your fee.

Your bank may be prepared to give you an overdraft facility on your existing account or offer you a small business loan based upon your business plan.

Alternatively, you may wish to consider a **Career Development Loan** (CDL). This is a deferred repayment loan scheme based upon an arrangement between the Department for Education and Employment and four major banks throughout Great Britain. It is designed to give you help to pay for vocational education or training providing the course you take is over a period of less than 2 years. A CDL, subject to approval, may allow you to borrow enough money to cover up to 80 per cent of your course fees plus all costs of essential books, material and course expenses including travel. You can apply whether you are employed or unemployed and you do not have to be an account holder at one of the four banks involved in the scheme. The repayments commence three months after the completion of your course, thus allowing you a period to get trained and established. Your application will require a business plan. Further details are included in the Useful Addresses and Resource Guide.

If you have been unemployed prior to undertaking your training, you may be eligible for an allowance to help you get started in your business.

If you are currently employed and are wishing to utilise your new aromatherapy skills within your existing occupation (such as nursing or sports therapy), you may be able to receive funding from your employer.

Approaching the bank manager

If you choose to apply for a loan or overdraft facility, a visit to your bank manager will be required. In many people's minds, the image of a bank manager is a distorted one! Remember that the manager is there to run the bank at a profit. If your manager believes your plans will succeed and help him in his job, then he is likely to approve your application. Here are some tips to help improve your chances:

● Plan ahead. Do not leave it until the last minute to apply for a loan or overdraft.

● Telephone to make an appointment in good time and send in a copy of your business plan in advance of your meeting.

● At the meeting itself, convey confidence and commitment, and supply evidence that you have considered your future plans with care and attention to detail.

● Be prepared to answer questions.

If all goes well, you can proceed with paying for your course. If you are refused a loan, you will need to evaluate why this may have happened.

(a) It may be simply that this particular bank is unwilling to invest in small businesses, in which case you should approach other banks.

(b) It may be that your business plan lacked detail. If so, ask yourself how it may be improved.

(c) It may be that what you have proposed is not financially viable. If this is the case, re-think your plans and seek professional advice.

Negotiating payment with your college

Having now secured the means to pay for your course, you may find that your college has several payment options. Normally, a non-refundable proportion of the fee is paid at enrolment followed by either the remainder on commencement or payment by instalments. Previous qualifications may exempt you from certain parts of your course. In such cases, the fee should be adjusted accordingly. If the college's normal scheme of payment is not possible for you, try and negotiate another means of payment. Many colleges are prepared to make an exception to their routine, providing the full course fee is guaranteed.

Using your student status

An additional student benefit that is often under-utilised is your entitlement to a range of reductions upon production of evidence that you are a student. Some essential oil suppliers and bookshops offer considerable student discounts as do some high street shops. Other 'perks' include reductions on transport costs and theatre tickets. Ask your college to provide you with a student 'card' or letter confirming your student status.

SUMMARY

The concepts of healing and essential oils may initially seem incompatible with dealing bluntly with finances. Yet in order to be a competent therapist, you will need to be an effective manager of your own affairs. This chapter has helped you:

● appreciate the need for developing a business sense

● realistically assess and calculate your worth

● budget for your new venture

● prepare a business plan

● apply for financial assistance to pay for your training.

Chapter 4 helps you to adjust to the role of being a student aromatherapist.

CASE STUDIES

Jane steps into full commitment

Jane's previous job as a bank clerk has helped her to appreciate the value of careful budgeting and financial planning. She opts for a Career Development Loan to fund her course and prepares a business plan accordingly. She discovers that the prices charged by other aromatherapists in her area vary quite considerably and she decides to book a few treatments for herself in the interests of 'market research'.

Theresa chooses to progress at her own pace

Theresa can afford to pay for her own training but decides to progress gradually rather than commit to a full aromatherapy course. She enrols on an introductory course in aromatherapy in her local area. She is informed that if she then decides to progress onto the full course, the cost of the introductory sessions will be deducted and her payments for the full course may be spread over the course period. She is not concerned about making a business plan or calculating her fees as her prime motivation for studying aromatherapy is not financial and she is unsure of how she will ultimately use her skills.

Mark takes advantage of his contacts and skills

Mark is interested in the adult education course in aromatherapy run at the leisure centre, particularly as he is entitled to a reduction in its cost. He is already exempt from parts of the course because of his existing skills and qualifications. He thus decides to apply for a small overdraft facility to help pay for the course expenses. He is comfortable about charging clients for his treatments and has decided to increase his existing fees to include the additional costs with prior notification to his clients.

THINKING IT THROUGH

1. Ask yourself how you can build a healthy attitude towards money whilst retaining a caring nature as a therapist.

2. Make a list of the people in your locality who will be able to give you independent financial advice.

3. How do your proposed fees compare to those charged by others in your locality? What factors have most influenced your price?

4

Being a Student

One of the big challenges of entering a training environment as an adult is that of re-acquaintance with the concepts of study, discipline and group dynamics. As a mature student, you may not have actively studied for years. This chapter aims to assist you with understanding the key differences between adult and compulsory education. It offers practical guidance as to how to develop study skills to gain maximum benefit from your chosen course.

GOING BACK TO SCHOOL

There are five basic factors that differentiate adult learning from your experiences of compulsory education. It is important to fully grasp these differences as they will help you adapt to your student role more easily.

1. It is your choice to enter training. This means your motivation is sufficient for you to engage both time and money in study. As you will see, motivation dictates how much you get out of your course. Most mature students expect to work hard!

2. Your decision to train has been made with a clear goal in mind: to become an aromatherapist. This means that your training is going to equip you with skills you intend to make use of in the immediate future.

3. You are entering the learning environment with a wealth of life experience from which you can draw upon to enrich your learning.

4. Your fellow students will be similarly motivated and bring with them a rich collection of experience and social skills. They will contribute as much to your course as the tutors.

5. Last, but no less important is the fact that you are an adult. This

means your relationships with the tutors will be different from those you had with teachers at school.

Understanding the learning process

It is recognised (Heron, 1981 – see Further Reading) that there are three main types of knowledge that go towards making up an individual:

1. *Propositional* – briefly, this form of knowledge is to do with facts and theory and is often delivered by straight lecturing or reading set texts.

2. *Practical* – this form of knowledge is concerned with the acquisition of practical skills but does not necessarily encourage you to divert from the set way in which to act. A good example of this is learning a basic massage sequence for the first time.

3. *Experiential* – this form of knowledge comes from putting into practice your theory and new skills and learning through reflection and previous experience. It is basically *learning* through *doing*.

Questions and answers

Which of these forms of learning did I experience at school?
It is likely that you received mainly propositional and practical learning opportunities at school. Although school education styles have changed considerably over the years, as an adult, you may have recollections of long lessons delivered by the teacher with little opportunity to act, question or reflect on the subject. Your experiences of practical sessions are likely to have involved highly structured forms of guidance and supervision.

Which of these forms is more suited to adult learning?
If your training values your previous skills and experiences and encourages you to learn through a practical, active and reflective approach, this indicates an experiential form of learning. Adult learning is generally more suited to this approach. This does not mean there will not be propositional or practical forms on your course. These will often form the underpinning knowledge for your experiential learning process.

Why is it that many aromatherapy colleges prefer students over 21 years of age?
As aromatherapy is a person-centered discipline, a degree of maturity is

considered an essential quality of the therapist. This maturity usually comes with life experience. It is unusual to find fully mature students straight from school. However, most colleges select prospective students on their individual merits and will consider applications by younger persons.

Experiential learning style

This style of training may be unfamiliar to you. Experiential learning usually involves less formal lecturing, more work conducted in groups, more role play, discussion and the opportunity for personal growth and development. It demands that you participate in your own learning process and refine and modify your learning through direct application and experience. For some people used to a more 'structured' form of training, this can feel awkward at first.

In traditional teaching/learning structures, the tutor assumes the active role, 'dispensing' information whilst the student more often than not is a relatively passive recipient. In adult education, this situation is often reversed. The tutors respect your previous experiences and motivation. Their role is more as **facilitators** for your studies than leaders. In fact, they may well be younger than you and have less life experience! Additionally, you need to understand that your course is *your* responsibility. It is unusual for tutors in adult education to be chasing you for homework and assignments. It is expected that your motivation and desire to succeed will ensure you keep up with your studies. Figure 6 outlines the three components of the experiential learning process.

Setting ground rules

Experiential learning usually carries with it an element of risk and personal challenge. It demands that you become actively engaged in your own learning process. Thus the course becomes very personal to

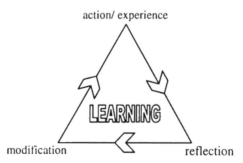

Fig. 6. The process of experiential learning.

you. This is particularly the case in aromatherapy training. For example:

(a) You will be experiencing how the aroma of essential oils affects the mood and emotions.

(b) You will discover how the power of touch has profound psychophysiological consequences.

(c) You will learn how to work with others on a deep and personal level.

(d) You may find that the course becomes a catalyst for your own personal growth and development.

All these factors will heighten the intensity and your involvement in the subject. For you to truly learn, you must allow it to become part of your life experience. This can be painful as well as rewarding. You therefore need the close support and total acceptance of your fellow students, who in turn will need the same from you. It is often helpful to bring this to the attention of the whole group at the start of the course, so that together, you can devise and agree upon a set of ground rules to which you all try to adhere for the duration of the course. Such ground rules may include that the class:

- respects each other's individuality
- allows the safety and freedom to express emotion
- respects each other's dignity during practical sessions
- gives mutual support and encouragement
- respects confidentiality
- retains an atmosphere of openness, trust and honesty.

MAKING THE MOST OF YOUR COURSE

Irrespective of how long or short your course, 'time always flies' and many students are caught out by the speed and depth of the course and fall behind with their studies. To take full advantage of your learning environment, you need to be well prepared, enthusiastic and resourceful from the moment you register.

Counting on motivation
Your level of motivation dictates how much you gain. Constantly

remind yourself of your initial reasons for undertaking training and keep your enthusiasm and good humour throughout. There will undoubtedly be periods during the course when you question your ability; most students go through an 'I know nothing at all' phase! Desire to succeed. Have a mental image of yourself after your course, practising aromatherapy successfully.

Gaining the upper hand

Most professional colleges supply the syllabus/timetable in advance of the course start date. Usually, a recommended reading list is provided at the same time. Use the period *before* your course begins to familiarise yourself with the subjects to be taught and start preparatory reading. Once the course begins, use the timetable to prepare in advance for each class. This will allow you more time to truly *listen* to the tutor rather than struggling to grasp key concepts when they are newly presented.

Using your resources

Here are a few pointers to using resources to maximise your learning opportunities.

Asking the boss!

Course tutors are a resource that many students under-utilise. They are there to give you guidance, support and advice. By asking relevant questions, you are indicating your level of engagement and many tutors will be happy to supply you with further support and information outside the class. Whenever you have a query, note it down as it arises and wait for the right opportunity for clarification. This may be during class time or during your own home study periods. If not noted down, questions often go unasked and therefore unanswered.

Getting out the books

Many colleges have an extensive library relevant to the subjects you are studying. Reading around your subject broadens your understanding.

Using the tools of the trade

Start using your essential oils from the first day of class. Having budgeted for them, you now need to utilise them as they greatly enhance your understanding and experience of the subject. Regularly handle and smell your oils, making notes of your impressions and results.

Growing herbs

If you have a garden, it is simple and fun to grow essential oil bearing plants to assist you with your studies. Plants such as thyme, rosemary, peppermint, clary sage and lavender are widely available in plant nurseries and can add a new dimension to your learning experience.

Practising your skills
Incorporate your new knowledge and skills from the first day. Involve your family and friends in your study of anatomy and physiology and find willing 'bodies' on which to practise your massage. In short, as already noted, make this course a part of your life. In this way, you will gain the maximum rewards.

Going for treatment
While studying, a particularly useful experience is to have regular professional aromatherapy treatments from others. This is of benefit to you personally and gives you a good perspective on what it is like to be a client. Be prepared to learn from yourself. Record and reflect on all your experiences.

Putting on your therapist's hat
Step into the professional image of a therapist from day one. Dress appropriately for class, and use the duration of the course to find and adapt to an image you feel most comfortable with as a therapist. This takes a degree of experimentation; something best done in the safe realm of your class with peer support than left until the launch of your career. More information regarding image is found in Chapter 6.

GETTING ORGANISED

In order to incorporate all aspects of your course into one cohesive whole, it is necessary to develop a disciplined study strategy and method. Here are a few pointers to get you started.

Preparing to study
Remember that the key to successful learning is **active involvement**. This takes time and energy but is always fruitful. Consider the examples of active learning in Table 6.

Disciplining yourself
Having made the commitment to study, the next step is to allow the time and opportunity to fulfil your aims and aspirations. Discipline is an essential part of getting organised. Look carefully at your syllabus and

Table 6. Examples of active learning opportunities

having regular aromatherapy treatments
allocating regular time for study
taking part in role play activities
keeping records of experiences
sitting in on professional treatment sessions
working in a supervised clinic setting
being open to personal growth
smelling essential oils regularly
making blends of oils for different conditions
listening to the tutor
comparing notes with fellow students
being prepared to reflect on your experiences
    and modify your actions
compiling an aromatherapy dossier of articles
    and product information

timetable and construct your own personal study regime. The time you allocate for each subject should be in direct proportion to the amount of time spent in class, rather than in relation to the amount of *your* interest or preference.

Night owl or early bird?
Everyone has his or her own optimum time for concentration and freshness. Ascertain which part of the day is best for you. The number of hours of study per week will be dictated by the particular course you choose; your tutor will be able to advise you on the recommended minimum home study time. The secret is to make your study periods an integral part of your course rather than unwelcome chores.

The ideal study environment
As far as possible, ensure your place of study is conducive to the task; adequate lighting, warmth, supportive chair and table, and textbooks within reach are your minimum requirements. Freedom from interruption and noise are also desirable and may need careful explanation and planning with members of the household. If your home environment is not conducive to study, consider working at your local library or the college itself.

Making notes

Writing things down is an essential part of your learning experience. It has been said that 'writing is a crucial step without which learning is incomplete'. The very act of writing internalises your newly acquired knowledge.

Every student has a personal style of writing and making notes. Rediscover or develop your own method early on in the course and maintain this style consistently throughout.

There are three main reasons for note-making:

1. *As an aid to your concentration.* By writing down key points as you hear/read them, you follow what is being taught.

2. *As an aid to your understanding.* Making notes helps you consolidate points and makes them available in your own words.

3. *To provide a record.* Note-making is helpful for further study and revision. Your preliminary notes will be subjected to several stages of elaboration, revision and condensation.

Keeping it legible

Your notes need to be legible and in your own words rather than copied directly from text or verbatim from lectures. This is the art of 'making' notes as opposed to 'taking' notes. The learning process through making notes involves participating in the lesson by listening, watching or reading, followed by thought/reflection, eliciting key points from the subject and then putting into your own words your understanding. This is a continuous process and follows the same steps as illustrated in Figure 6.

The form your notes take is unique to you. Some students use abbreviations for common words or phrases. If you do so, ensure you are consistent with these abbreviations to avoid frustration later when you come to read through what you have written. You may prefer to use diagrams, flowcharts or lists instead of text. Colour coding topics or key points may also be helpful. As long as your notes are organised and make sense to you, there is no right or wrong format.

For these reasons, you will understand why using other students' notes to 'catch up' on class or work you have missed is not reliable; you are merely reading their interpretation of the subject, in their unique language and style which may differ widely from your own.

Tips on essay writing

Essays:

- organise your thoughts and incorporate your knowledge gained in class with previous experience and private study

- help you deepen your understanding of the subject and focus your awareness on key points

- provide your tutor with evidence of your level of understanding

- make excellent revision aids.

When required to write an essay, bear in mind the need to keep within the parameters set by the title and depth required by the tutor. Understand the question and answer it precisely, having given it plenty of thought *before* putting pen to paper. Every essay should consist of at least five parts:

1. *Title* – as given to you by the tutor.

2. *Introduction* – state clearly the purpose of the essay and the course the essay will take. This is usually no more than a paragraph in length.

3. *Main text* – the body of the essay where you explore all points necessary to fulfil the title. The length of the main text is dependent on the depth required.

4. *Summary and conclusion* – reiterate the key points you have made in the text and close the essay.

5. *References* – it is professional and useful for revision purposes to note at the end of the essay the sources of reference you have used.

Using study aids

Some students find it helpful to record the lectures they attend on cassette. This leaves them free to listen and make loose notes during the class itself. They are then able to playback at a later time and make further notes. Whilst this may appear useful in principle, it is wise to remember there may be technical hitches to this practice! In addition, not all establishments or tutors permit recording of class sessions; check first to avoid embarrassment to either yourself or the tutor.

Other study aids available include anatomy and physiology wall charts and models, aromatherapy posters and revision cards. You may find these advertised in the therapy journals listed in the Useful Addresses and Resource Guide.

Learning about essential oils

In your course, a number of essential oils will be studied in depth. The thought of being able to retain all the necessary information can be a daunting prospect to even the most enthusiastic student!

A useful study aid is to create your own essential oil profile for each essential oil. Many students use a large or medium-size card index filing system. On the card profile, the key points about the essential oil are listed together with a summary of key therapeutic information. You may leave space on each card to record your own uses/experiences/ observations. By putting them into an accessible format, the profiles may be used readily for revision and reference purposes. An example of a typical essential oil card index is shown in Figure 7.

Learning Latin names

Learning the Latin names of plants that produce essential oils is a difficult but necessary part of being an aromatherapist. To facilitate learning, make a habit of referring to essential oils by their correct botanic name from day one.

Taking time out

Whilst your course will occupy a great deal of your time, it is important to acknowledge that you also require adequate rest and relaxation! If you have a partner or family, it is important to spend quality time together. Ideally, plan for one full day per week where work is neither discussed nor undertaken. This nourishes your relationships and home life and enables you to recommence your studies with a fresh and new perspective.

NETWORKING WITH FELLOW STUDENTS

The contribution of your fellow students is a key feature of adult education. During your course you will learn much from one another and may form close working relationships that last long after your course has ended. Do not underestimate your individual contribution to the group as a whole.

Sharing knowledge and resources

Working on projects and homework together can be a valuable learning experience as each person contributes a slightly differing perspective on

Front of card

LATIN NAME	EUCALYPTUS GLOBULUS
Common name	Eucalyptus
Botanical Family	Myrtaceae
Part of plant used	leaves and young twigs
Method of extraction	steam Distillation
Country of origin	Spain and Portugal are main producers
Key Chemistry	oxide (1,8-cineole up to 70%), terpenes (e.g. pinene, limonene)
Key therapeutic action	e.o. for RESPIRATORY TRACT
Other uses	expectorant, decongestant, antiseptic, febrifuge - use for: sinusitis, 'flu, bronchial problems. Mildly diuretic analgesic, rubefacient, antirheumatic cephalic, mentally stimulating
Safety information	can irritate if used in the bath

Rear of card

Aroma characteristics	sweet, penetrating, medicinal –'Vicks vaporub'
Blending information	strong aroma, piercing – use small amounts. Blends well with herbaceous e.o.'s, woods, resins. Less well with floral
Methods of application	inhalations/ compresses/ ointments/ massage/ not for bathing
Personal notes:	
20/11/ox	2 drops Euc. glob. with 2 drops Ros. off. in steam inhalation for 'flu - good effect.
25/11/ox	Blend Euc. glob. (3), Junip. com. (4) and Lav. off. (6) in 25mls almond oil for Mum's arthritic knee. Next time try stronger blend.
1/12/ox	Inhaled Euc. glob. from tissue for blocked sinus. Rapid relief.

Fig. 7. Typical essential oil profile on a card index file.

the subject studied. This enhances and enriches your appreciation and understanding. 'Brain storming' and sharing of resources such as books or anatomical models is a distinct advantage of working with others.

Practice makes perfect

Practising your new skills is an indispensable part of learning. Your expertise and confidence will grow quickly with regular practice. By working with your peers, you not only have the opportunity to practise your skills in a secure environment, but also have the advantage of 'expert' feedback on technique and treatment approach. Role play is a form of experiential learning. It helps you to develop your interpersonal skills in a safe environment. Examples of skills you can practise with your peers include:

● introducing yourself

● explaining what a treatment involves

● explaining fees and accepting payment

● taking a consultation

● recording treatment and findings

● practising listening skills

● assisting with de-robing and maintaining modesty

● selecting and blending essential oils

● mastering massage techniques and sequences

● refining your sense of smell

● designing forms and promotional literature.

Respecting individuality

As a group member, do not lose sight of your own individuality or that of others. Everyone has a basic need for personal space and this applies irrespective of whether you are in a group or alone. There will be times when you have differences of opinion or feel uncomfortable relating to certain persons in the class. This is a normal part of group dynamics and can provide a constructive learning opportunity.

GAINING VALUABLE PRACTICE

Working on yourself

Most students commence by working on themselves to appreciate the potential uses of aromatherapy. This enhances your learning as you 'experiment' with different blends and applications. This makes your work real to you and consolidates your learning. Make a record of all your experiments, observations and experiences as you go along.

Working on others

Once you have mastered the basics and are starting to gain confidence with your peer practice sessions, you may consider working on your family and friends. This adds greatly to your experience, as you will be entering a more realistic work setting.

Initially, relatives and friends may have difficulty adapting to your new role as a therapist. You may find they appear not to take your studies seriously to begin with. It will be up to you to explain clearly your new role and be consistent in your approach to treatment. Many people know very little about aromatherapy; it will be part of your role to provide more information. Talk to them about what aromatherapy entails — remember that their understanding may be very different from yours. Common misconceptions you may encounter include:

- 'aromatherapy involves sniffing perfumes out of bottles'

- 'aromatherapy is a pamper therapy'

- 'only women have aromatherapy'

- 'massage has sleazy connotations'.

If you do not succeed in helping your family and friends to adapt to your new therapeutic image, it will be difficult to work with them and give them the deep long-lasting effects you desire. If you are successful, your relatives and friends will become an important source of support and promotion when you qualify. Word of mouth is your surest form of advertising.

Charging for treatments

Charging for treatments raises many issues for the would-be therapist. The answer lies with you as an individual. It can be useful to practise charging and accepting payment before you qualify, particularly if you identified negative attitudes towards money in Chapter 3. However, if you have student aromatherapy insurance (generally available through your college), you may find that the cover is valid only if you do *not* make a charge for your treatment.

SUMMARY

Becoming a student and adapting to adult learning strategies is a challenging aspect of your training. This chapter has helped you to:

● identify the key learning strategies for the mature student

● develop a disciplined study approach to your course

● consider the impact of fellow students during your training

● maximise all your learning opportunities.

CASE STUDIES

Jane throws herself into her studies

An organised and disciplined person by nature, Jane quickly establishes an effective study routine. She enjoys the mental challenge of the factual subjects but is finding the practical and group sessions more difficult. She is impatient to learn but unaccustomed to working with her hands. As she is studying on the full-time course, she is aware that she will not have much opportunity to practise her skills outside college. As Jane is determined to make aromatherapy her full-time career, she does not mind studying hard and is inclined to work every day at the expense of her leisure time.

Theresa adjusts to her student role

Soon after commencing the course, Theresa is struggling with the volume of work expected of her. Having not studied for many years, she is finding it difficult to establish a regular working pattern despite having the time and ideal working environment at home. Aware that this will adversely affect her studies, she approaches her tutor for advice. Together, they establish a formal home study plan for Theresa to follow. In class, she finds it hard to listen and make adequate notes. Her tendency is to try and write down everything she hears and subsequently loses the thread of the lesson. She prefers the practical and group sessions and as one of the older students, she offers much valuable advice and support.

Mark tries to combine work and play

Finding the time to study is hard for Mark as he feels tired at the end of each day's work at the gym. He is enthusiastic about the course, has adapted well to the practical sessions and is already seeing how his new skills will benefit his clients. He records each evening class on his minicorder and plays the tape on his way to and from work. His notes are minimal and mainly consist of sketches, lists and flowcharts to highlight key points. His weekends are mostly spent with sporting friends who tease him about his studies. He is at a loss as to how to convince them that learning aromatherapy will augment his professional skills.

THINKING IT THROUGH

1. What risk is Jane running with her committed approach to studying? How might she avoid this happening?

2. How may Theresa engage the help of her fellow students in order to master her grasp of the theoretical parts of her course?

3. What can Mark do to lessen the lighthearted approach to his studies from his friends?

5

Sourcing the Tools of the Trade

The art and science of aromatherapy is reliant on the knowledge and skills of the therapist plus the quality of the products used. Bombarded with the enormous and astonishing range of aromatherapy products available on the market, you may initially feel unsure of how to find a supplier that meets your individual needs. This chapter is concerned with helping you to find reputable suppliers of quality equipment and products.

ASSESSING WHAT IS NEEDED

There are several 'tools of the trade' that are necessary to acquire in order to study and to practise aromatherapy. The two main tools that are the most important and costly are:

1. massage couch and linen
2. essential oils and related products.

If you are applying for a loan or creating a business plan, be sure to include the costs of these essential items in your calculations.

Gathering information

The first thing to do is create a dossier of information together with current price lists. The classified sections of popular and professional health magazines commonly carry adverts for couch and essential oil companies. Ask around fellow students, massage therapists and aromatherapists for their suppliers' names and details. Health fairs and exhibitions are good places to visit to locate and talk to prospective suppliers. This also gives you the opportunity to try out the tools before you buy. Your college may also carry information and supply a range of oils and related products.

Locating reliable suppliers

Once you start to compile a dossier, you will quickly discover there are a whole range of equipment, products and essential oil suppliers to choose from. It can be difficult in the beginning to discern which supplier is going to best meet your needs as a professional aromatherapist. The following advice will help you identify your precise requirements.

MAKING THE RIGHT CHOICES

Choosing your massage couch

Also called a table or plinth, your massage couch is a long-lasting investment for your business. It is thus essential that it conforms to your needs perfectly. It must be robust, and easy to clean and maintain. It must not creak or squeak! You may wish to check that the manufacturer gives a guarantee that covers defects, maintenance and repair.

Figure 8 outlines six factors to consider in choosing a massage couch.

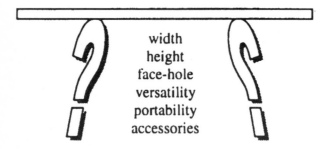

width
height
face-hole
versatility
portability
accessories

Fig. 8. Choosing a massage couch.

1. *Is width important?* Some therapists prefer wide couches for client comfort. Whilst being pleasing to the client, a wider couch adds to its weight and may make carrying difficult. Most couch companies provide couches of differing widths.

2. *Does the height need to be adjustable?* If you are not the sole user of the massage couch or if you practise a number of therapies needing the couch at different heights, a hydraulic couch or one with adjustable legs will be necessary. A couch of the right height promotes good technique, minimises fatigue and reduces the risk of injury.

3. *Does it need to be portable?* If so, it will need to be a folding model of a weight that you can manage without strain. Although more costly, couches with aluminium frames are lighter than those made from wood. A mobile therapist will also require a durable fitted carrying case to protect the couch in transit. If you plan to use your existing car for home visiting, be sure to check that a couch will fit in it!

4. *Does it need to be versatile?* If you practise more than one therapy, you may need a couch that has a range of functions. For example, a raising section may be needed for treatments such as reflexology or facial treatments.

5. *Does it need a face-hole?* In theory, a face-hole permits the client to lie prone and breathe comfortably without the need for turning their head to the side. This is a personal choice as not all clients appreciate using one. A face hole is usually an optional extra that needs to be requested. Some manufacturers provide a 'plug' to fit in the face hole if it is not required.

6. *Do I need accessories?* Bolsters, face-rings, fitted couch covers and other accessories are often available from the couch manufacturer. To have matching equipment and accessories can help convey a professional image. You may be able to make your own at a lower cost.

Buying secondhand

From time to time, there is the opportunity to buy secondhand massage couches through advertisements in journals and local papers. Whilst the cost may be considerably lower than a new couch, bear in mind that it should still meet your needs as explained above.

Choosing your essential oil supplier

Most essential oil suppliers for professional aromatherapists operate by mail order. Few sell direct to the public in high street shops. It may take you several small orders from various suppliers before deciding on the ones that meet your needs.

There are numerous suppliers on the market, providing essential oils of variable quality. It is important to find a source of consistently high quality essential oils for your work. These will be obtained at considerable expense. Buying essential oils is not an area where cost cutting is advised. You generally get the quality that you pay for. If you buy and use sub-standard or adulterated products, you run the risk of not only minimising the efficacy of your treatment but also provoking negative health reactions with your clients.

Figure 9 lists nine questions to ask yourself when looking for an essential oil supplier.

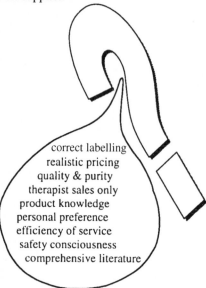

correct labelling
realistic pricing
quality & purity
therapist sales only
product knowledge
personal preference
efficiency of service
safety consciousness
comprehensive literature

Fig. 9. Choosing an essential oil supplier.

1. *Do they deal solely with professional aromatherapists?* If they do, they are more likely to anticipate your needs as a therapist and provide quality essential oils and related products. They may also give student and practitioner discounts.

2. *Do they provide a comprehensive catalogue and price list?* This should include at least the full botanical names of the plants, their country of origin, method of extraction and part of the plant that the oil was obtained from. Information should also be available concerning the company and its commitment to quality.

3. *Can they give you assurances regarding quality and purity?* As tampering and adulteration of these products is so widespread, it is becoming increasingly important to ascertain the quality of the essential oils you buy. You need to be confident that your supplier is doing all in their power to ensure you have access to pure essential oils. An increasing number of suppliers are now subjecting their

essential oils to independent analysis to determine purity and give assurance regarding quality. They should be happy to pass this information on to you. A reputable supplier will have a system whereby they monitor the quality of their products, store and bottle them under controlled conditions and have a regular turnover of stock. Do not be afraid to demand what methods of quality assurance they employ.

4. *Are their products clearly and correctly labelled?* Pure essential oils are always sold in dark glass bottles and each bottle of essential oil should clearly identify the common name and botanical name of the plant, together with safety information such as 'keep away from children' and 'not to be taken internally'. The presence of a batch number is essential; it suggests the company may have in place some form of quality control. In the UK, the Aromatherapy Trade Council has established guidelines for safety, labelling and packaging of essential oils and works closely with Trading Standards officers. Their members consist mainly of essential oil suppliers that adhere to their code of practice. A list of their members is available. See Useful Addresses and Resource Guide.

5. *Are they safety conscious?* Most reputable suppliers provide integral dropper inserts on their bottles. These regulate the drops of essential oil from the bottle and have the advantage of acting as a safety device to prevent accidental ingestion. Additionally, some professional suppliers will seek to establish the qualification of the buyer before selling particular essential oils that have contraindications to their use.

6. *Are they knowledgeable about their essential oils?* Reputable suppliers have an in-depth knowledge about their products and should be happy to answer your queries.

7. *Is their service prompt and efficient?* The efficiency of a company often reflects their commitment to their work. If your orders repeatedly arrive late, incomplete or badly packaged, you may begin to have doubts as to the quality of the product.

8. *Are their prices realistic?* You will soon become familiar with the variable price ranges of essential oils. Be wary of a supplier whose prices never vary and who sells expensive essential oils for a considerable reduction in price compared to other companies. This is where your dossier will become extremely helpful in order to compare prices offered. Elaborate packaging can significantly add to the cost

of the essential oil itself; ask yourself if you are paying for the design and aesthetic appearance rather than the quality of the oil inside the bottle.

9. *Do you like the essential oils they are selling?* At the end of the day, you are likely to select your supplier not only on the above details but also on whether you appreciate the aroma and qualities of the oils they provide. This is an important and highly personal aspect of locating a supplier; with practice, you will acquire a 'nose' that will help you compare essential oils from different companies.

Extending your product range

As you progress through your course and gain more knowledge and skills, you will seek other related products to enhance your care. These may include:

- hydrolats or hydrosols
- creams and lotions
- gels
- soaps
- diffusers
- dispersing agents
- vegetable base oils
- shampoo/shower bases.

Your essential oil supplier may have all or most of these products in their range.

AVOIDING COMMON MISTAKES

Being hasty

Do not rush into acquiring your tools of the trade. You need to choose with care and experience. In the interim period, you can always improvise with working on a firm bed or the floor until you have the massage couch that meets your needs. Your college may also supply essential oils and other products such as uniforms and paper couch rolls. This can be a useful and convenient (though possibly more costly) way to obtain the items you need whilst you are studying, giving you the time to seriously research a supplier elsewhere.

Using and storing

Essential oils and vegetable base oils are perishable commodities. Once they begin to degrade, you cannot halt the process and they may become ineffective or harmful to use with your clients. Thus, once you have found a supplier, do not be tempted to buy large stocks of essential oils, particularly in the early stages of your training and career. Start with a minimum number of essential oils in 5, 10 or 15 ml quantities and increase the range of oils gradually as your course progresses. Keep your essential oils stored:

● properly sealed

● in small glass bottles

● in a cool, dark place

● away from children and pets.

If you do buy an essential oil in a quantity larger than 15 ml, you may wish to decant it into several smaller dark glass bottles to reduce the headspace of air above the oil's surface. This will help protect against oxidation.

Many therapists mark the date they first open the bottle on the label. This gives them some idea of the oil's potential shelf life.

Vegetable base oils have a variable shelf life dependent upon their degree of refinement and fatty acid composition. Buy only amounts that you will need for a few months and store them in a cool place with a minimum of headspace of air.

Accepting gifts

When you enter the world of aromatherapy, your family and friends will undoubtedly seize upon the opportunity to buy you gifts of oils and related products. If you do not specify precisely your needs, you may receive well-intentioned gifts of low quality products due to the explosion of 'aromatherapy' products on the market. With a bit of education and a few hints, you can point them in the direction of reputable quality products that will be extremely useful to you in your training and career.

SUMMARY

Buying quality essential oils and equipment for your practice is a costly enterprise that directly impacts on the quality of your work and client interaction. This chapter has encouraged you to:

- get access to the tools of the trade

- consider carefully your massage couch requirements

- ask the right questions to find an essential oil supplier

- think ahead to related products you may need in the future

- avoid common and costly mistakes.

CASE STUDIES

Jane gets help from her college

Upon enrolment, Jane is informed that a massage couch supplier will visit the college to present its range of equipment and accessories to her aromatherapy class later in the term. She decides to wait for this visit before making her final choice. In the meantime, she has started to collect various brochures and price lists for comparison and is working on different height couches in class to find the best level for her stature. She bought a starter kit of essential oils from the college and has already begun to 'experiment' with them at home.

Theresa takes things slowly

As Theresa is unsure of her long-term future as a therapist, she is unwilling to make a serious financial commitment by buying a massage couch at this early stage. She therefore decides to improvise by placing padding on a table at home and finds this a suitable substitute for the time being. She already has a range of essential oils that she bought in various high street locations and has become aware of their variable quality. On the recommendation of her aromatherapist, she has taken steps to source essential oils from a mail order supplier of quality essential oils.

Mark uses his existing tools and contacts

One of Mark's biggest investments as a sports therapist was to purchase a fixed, hydraulic massage couch with numerous adaptable features for use in his clinic at the leisure centre. He also has a portable couch for on-site work that he rarely uses. He offers to lend the latter to one of his fellow aromatherapy students until they find one of their own. His supplier of therapeutic products such as gels and creams is also able to supply vegetable base oils but he needs to locate a supplier of quality essential oils. He finds a few addresses in his health magazine and uses them as a starting point for further research

THINKING IT THROUGH

1. Why are essential oils so variable in price and what factors contribute to their overall cost?

2. What are the properties and qualities of a vegetable base that you consider important for aromatherapy massage?

3. Why is it that most essential oil suppliers for professional aromatherapists rarely sell to the general public via high street outlets?

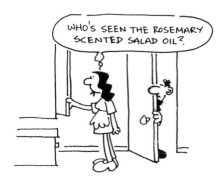

6

Preparing Your Niche

You do not have to wait to receive your aromatherapy qualification before starting to publicise your skills and attract clients. Much can be prepared in advance to ensure that you will reap the benefits of a successful career. Preparing the ground well and sowing seeds directly affects the harvest itself! This chapter aims to give you tips and encouragement to work towards your goal whilst you are still completing your studies.

SURVEYING THE MARKET

Knowing your potential client base

In order to attract clients, you first need to ascertain the type of client you are most likely to treat.

Ask yourself . . .

1. Who will want aromatherapy in my area?
2. How many people are likely to want my treatments?
3. Why would they be coming?
4. How often would they come?
5. How many treatments would they have?
6. What would they be prepared to pay?
7. How can I attract them?

Answers to the above questions will depend very much upon the geographical location and the lifestyle of the local people. The image you project, the way in which you work and the publicity you make should take this into account. It is generally accepted that there are trends common to clients that attend for complementary therapies:

- 75 per cent of all people who go to mainstream complementary practitioners (excluding hypnotherapists) are aged 45 or over.

- over 65 per cent of them are women

- the average number of sessions they receive is three.

The reasons for attending aromatherapy treatments are extremely variable. A large majority of people attend for relaxation and help with a range of stress-related problems such as insomnia and anxiety; others attend for specific complaints such as pain control.

Many people pay for an aromatherapy treatment out of their **disposable income**, i.e. money they have set aside for non-essential expenses. The amount of disposable income a person has varies according to general geographical location and lifestyle. For example, if you are planning to offer treatments in an inner city area with high unemployment, your client base will be different from an aromatherapy practice in a wealthy suburb. Each area will have its own specific needs and problems that need addressing. You need to survey your area and decide on the best approach to attracting clients.

Ask yourself . . .
How might I adapt my services and means of attracting clients for working in

(a) an area of high disposable income

(b) an area of low disposable income

(c) a rural area

(d) an urban area.

Analysing other practices in the area

By visiting other aromatherapy clinics and talking with family and friends, you will soon build up certain impressions about the services already on offer in your locality. Find out what people like and dislike about individual clinics or treatments. Remember that the purpose is to assess different aspects of aromatherapy provision in the area, *not* to engage in active and unethical slander or poaching of clients from other practitioners! There is no reason why you should not study how other aromatherapists operate as long as you are not using the information to deceive or slander their work to others. This is purely an objective exercise that will help you plan how to create your own niche as an aromatherapist. It is helpful to extend this assessment to other natural health clinics in order to gain as broad an impression as possible.

Create a checklist for making an assessment of a clinic. Include all aspects, not just the treatment itself. Include, for example how welcome you were made to feel, the suitability of the premises, aspects of comfort, safety, hygiene and quality of promotional literature. From this information, you can decide how to improve upon the services that are available and avoid the mistakes of others.

Developing a specialist skill

In theory, there is always a niche for a specialist skill or different approach. This niche may not yet exist and will have to be created by you with a considerable amount of time and effort. What is extremely important is that the niche is suitable for the area you plan to work in. Location is extremely important; if you plan to be an aromatherapist specialising in baby massage and care of pregnant mothers, you are unlikely to be successful in an area with a population consisting mainly of persons over childbearing age! Examples of niches that already exist in the aromatherapy profession include combining essential oil use with:

● counselling

● hypnotherapy

● reflexology

● energy therapies such as Chakra balancing, healing and Reiki

● nursing or midwifery skills

● stress management

● on-site massage.

FINDING THE RIGHT IMAGE

Choosing what to wear

As a student, you are in the experimental process of adapting to your chosen role as an aromatherapist. This is the ideal time to find an image that most reflects who you are and the sort of client you are trying to attract. Above all, it is important that you feel comfortable with the image you are trying to project. Consider how your working image might be different in the following scenarios:

(a) in a beauty salon

(b) in a hospice environment

(c) visiting clients in their home

(d) in a hospital environment

(e) in a leisure centre

(f) in a high class health club

(g) in a wealthy area

(h) in a centre of drug and alcohol abuse.

For each of the above examples, ask yourself whether a formal or informal image would be most appropriate for attracting clients and helping them feel at ease. Try and form a mental picture of yourself in each of these roles.

What you wear needs to be practical as well as professional. For example, if you plan to visit people in their homes, bear in mind the amount of lifting and carrying of couches involved when choosing what to wear. Your clothing also needs to be machine washable, possibly to high temperatures in order to remove oil stains.

Remembering the bare minimum

No matter what image you choose, there are several essential points to remember:

- hair clean and free from your face

- fingernails unpainted and short

- minimum of make-up and distracting jewellery

- fresh, clean clothing

- good attention to personal hygiene

- absence of distracting perfume or after-shave

- fresh breath.

Considering other aspects of image

Image does not only include what you look like and the uniform/clothing you wear. It is also conveyed by the premises you work in, your manner, your business stationery and promotional literature. You need to ensure that your image is conveyed consistently across all these areas. Any discrepancy can confuse potential clients and put them off making appointments with you. Imagine the client, impressed by professional stationery and publicity, who makes an appointment and is met by a therapist in oil-stained clothing, with body odour and dirty fingernails!

Once you have found the image that suits you, stick to it. Clients appreciate uniformity. It helps them feel secure in their image of you and thus enables them to relax fully and focus on the treatment they receive. Do not make big changes to the professional image you project without serious consideration. That is why it is so helpful to experiment whilst you are still a student.

FORGING LINKS WITH OTHERS

Building bridges with other practitioners

In Chapter 1, you found that it is important to recognise your limits as a therapist, knowing you cannot be all things to all people. As a professional therapist, you need to have a referral system in place for when you are unable to meet the needs of your client. Making contact with other practitioners before you qualify and set up in practice is a valuable task. A knock-on effect from such contacts is that you establish a professional relationship with other practitioners who will be in a position to refer clients to you. Table 7 contains a comprehensive but not exhaustive list of practitioners you may wish to contact in your local area.

Trusting the opinions of others

Personal recommendations are very valuable when it comes to selecting therapists for client referral. Ask your family and friends for names of therapists they have felt happy with in the past. Otherwise, you may initially have to rely on local advertising and Yellow Pages to locate practitioners from different disciplines.

Once you have made a list, it is professional practice to write or telephone expressing the wish to meet, giving your reasons for doing so. Remember that the purpose is for you to meet and form an opinion as to whether you would feel comfortable referring a client to him or her.

Table 7. Practitioners of other disciplines

Doctor	Chiropodist	Osteopath
Naturopath	Fitness instructor	Reflexologist
Masseur	Sports therapist	Physiotherapist
Healer	Allergy specialist	Counsellor
Hypnotherapist	Acupuncturist	Medical Herbalist
Homeopath	Iridologist	Shiatsu practitioner
Chinese Herbalist	Chiropractor	Reiki practitioner
Nutritional	Cranio-sacral	Alexander
counsellor	therapist	practitioner

Most therapists will be pleased to find time to meet you as it may lead to increased appointments and widen their network of practitioners at the same time. They may also be happy for you to leave leaflets and/or business cards at their place of work.

In addition to finding other practitioners, it is useful to have the addresses and contact details of statutory support systems, local support groups and organisations. These may include:

● Citizens' Advice Bureau

● Relate (marriage guidance)

● Samaritans

● bereavement counsellors

● support structures such as Multiple Sclerosis Society

● Alcoholics Anonymous.

Your local advice centre will be able to provide a list of such contacts and addresses.

Networking for the future

Networking is an important aspect of your professionalism and survival as a therapist. Once your training is completed, you may suddenly feel very alone away from the camaraderie and support of fellow students. Those first few months can be a particularly difficult transition period. One way to ease yourself into being a fully-fledged aromatherapist is to maintain the support and friendship for as long a period as possible.

Before you leave college, ensure that you have some form of reunion arranged; some groups find a regular get-together to exchange news, views and experiences is particularly helpful.

Enquire in your local area if there are any groups interested in natural health that meet on a regular basis. This always provides an interesting forum for exchange of information and helps you to establish your role and position in the local area. Some pro-active groups organise speakers, from different disciplines – an ideal platform for you to make some publicity and educate others about aromatherapy. Chapter 7 provides basic guidelines on giving talks and demonstrations.

SOWING SEEDS FOR THE FUTURE

Preparing the ground

As a student, take every opportunity to prepare for the day when you have completed your course and are able to launch your career. The advance preparation such as building bridges with other professionals and creating a practitioner network will all help to ensure that people are aware of your services. Seek out opportunities to share with others what you are doing and explain what aromatherapy means to you.

Your obvious enjoyment and commitment to aromatherapy should come across in all communications with others. Even the most shy person can enthuse over a subject they feel strongly about.

Getting the right message across

In the early stages of eagerness, enthusiasm and excitement, it is easy to overestimate the potentials of your services. Remember that ethically you cannot diagnose, or claim or promise to cure. Your advertising should be discreet and not mislead the general public. You are now a representative of the aromatherapy profession. Thus you will need to convey the professionalism and seriousness of the therapy as well as the enthusiasm and wonderfulness of the art. Much of your time will be spent:

- educating others in the potentials of aromatherapy

- changing preconceptions regarding aromatherapy and massage

- creating the desire to try an aromatherapy treatment.

EVALUATING THE BEST WORKING APPROACH

Deciding how to use your skills

As an aromatherapist you have several options as to how you offer your services. Until recently, most aromatherapists chose to work as self-employed practitioners. As the profession has grown and gained in reputation, there are now increasing employment opportunities in different sectors. There are at least five options open to you for consideration:

1. working from home

2. home visiting

3. renting space in a clinic

4. leasing or buying your own premises

5. working for others.

You may wish to combine these options in order to suit the needs of your clients as well as yourself. For example, many therapists combine renting space in a clinic for a few days per week with home visiting for clients who cannot travel for the remainder.

For each working approach, there are advantages and disadvantages. You may wish to compile your own list to augment the points raised below.

Working from home

(See Table 8a.) One of the biggest challenges of working from home is balancing your home life with your professional work. It requires much commitment and self-discipline. Additionally, you will need to

Table 8a.   Working from home

Advantages	Disadvantages
Able to create the environment you wish	Difficult to separate work from home
No travelling expenses	Needs high commitment
Reduced overheads	Safety risk with strangers
Flexible working hours	May be liable for Capital Gains Tax

confirm that you are legally permitted to work from home. This will involve speaking with your landlord, building society or housing officer. Understanding neighbours are also vital! Be sure to inform them of what you plan to do.

Home visiting

Table 8b. Home visiting

Advantages	Disadvantages
Flexible working approach	Need reliable transport
Reduced overheads	Can get lost!
Client provides warmth and linen	More time-consuming per client
Client can rest immediately after treatment	Personal safety may be at risk

(See Table 8b.) Home visiting is an excellent option for those who neither have space at home nor wish to rent space in a clinic environment. However, the number of clients you see per day will be significantly reduced because of travelling time. Your fees will need to reflect this shortfall.

Renting clinic space

(See Table 8c.) If possible, choose to rent space in a clinic that already has a good reputation and a significant existing clientele. Ensure you

Table 8c. Renting clinic space

Advantages	Disadvantages
Clinic has an existing clientele	Rent subject to rise
Clinic has an existing profile in the community	Furnishings may not be to your liking
Advertising costs often shared	Appointments made by others
The opportunity to network with others	High overheads

feel at ease with the image the clinic projects as this will affect your clients' perceptions of your skills as a therapist. Don't be tempted to work in the clinic with the lowest rent without checking why this is the case.

Leasing your own premises

Table 8d.   Leasing or buying your own premises

Advantages	Disadvantages
Freedom to create your own business	High capital investment necessary
Can lease clinic space to other practitioners	More time managing than practising
Complete control of the business	Subject to higher rate of tax
Room for expanding your services	Ideal locations are most expensive

(See Table 8d.) Ensure you have expert and professional advice whenever considering leasing or buying premises. Both involve considerable expense. In the early stages, it may be wise to build a client base and firmly establish your role before considering such a commitment. You will need to identify any legal restrictions or necessary licences before making your decision.

Working for others

Table 8e.   Working for others

Advantages	Disadvantages
Guarantee of regular income	High client turnover – tiring
Publicity costs borne by employer	Standardised treatments expected
High client turnover – good experience	Salary/commission per client low
Employment may be abroad	Emphasis on product marketing

(See Table 8e.) When applying for a job as a therapist, it is essential to ascertain precisely your job description. Ensure that you do not sign any contract of employment without first having scrutinised all that is written with the help of a solicitor and having satisfied yourself that you can meet all the conditions laid down. The prospect of working abroad is particularly attractive to therapists; remember that you will also be more vulnerable to exploitation away from your home environment.

SUMMARY

Here are the main points explored in this chapter with regard to preparing your niche.

- Know your potential client base.

- Find out how to reach them.

- Make an assessment of the 'competition'.

- Decide on the image that marries your individuality with the profile of your clients.

- Create links with other professionals.

- Start generating interest in what you are doing.

- Select and explore the most appropriate working methods.

CASE STUDIES

Jane prepares in advance

With the aid of *Yellow Pages* and the local directory, Jane has prepared a list of aromatherapists operating within a 20-mile radius. She has drawn up a checklist of points she would like to assess regarding their practice and makes appointments with several to experience the quality of the treatments given. She has also started to approach other local practitioners such as chiropodist, physiotherapist and osteopath in order to compile a list of contacts. She has developed a good relationship with one of her fellow students; together they are considering renting space in a natural health clinic once they qualify.

Theresa is beginning to find her role

Theresa is already gaining valuable practice giving hand and foot massages to elderly family and friends. Witnessing the benefit they are receiving, she is spurred into thinking about developing her skills in an area where a mature and caring approach is required. As she is becoming increasingly involved with the work of her local hospice, Theresa is considering the possibility of offering her services there on a regular basis. To support her voluntary work, she has decided to dedicate one room of her home as a treatment room. She plans to receive paying clients who come recommended from friends and family.

Mark takes advantage of his speciality

As his aromatherapy course has progressed, Mark has become aware of the scarcity of sports therapists who practise aromatherapy. He decides to use this point to his advantage by speaking to members of his sports association and writing an article for their journal. He has also discovered how aromatherapy may enhance mood and reduce preperformance stress in his athletic clients and approaches the sports editor of his local paper with this unusual topic. They gladly agree to interview him and report on his progress over the coming year.

THINKING IT THROUGH

1. It has been found that more women attend for aromatherapy sessions than men. Why do you think this is the case and how might you attract a greater number of male clients?

2. Your image as a practitioner should encourage and give confidence to the type of client you are trying to attract. With regard to your own image, consider whether you are conveying the right signals to your proposed clientele.

3. It is recommended that you receive treatments from aromatherapists in your area for market research purposes. There is mixed opinion as to whether you should inform the therapist from the outset of your purposes for attending. What is your opinion?

7

Launching Your New Career

The previous chapters have encouraged you to think and plan ahead to the day when you are a qualified and practising aromatherapist. Now that day has arrived! Congratulate yourself and step confidently forward. This chapter discusses the realities and day-to-day practicalities of being a professional aromatherapist.

SETTLING INTO YOUR NEW ROLE

Making sure the hat fits

Having experimented as a student with your image and role, the time has now come to try it out 'for real'. The transition from student to fledgling aromatherapist is not an easy one; for some it can be quite a shock to be let loose in the big wide world!

Once you start treating members of the public, do not be afraid to tell them you are recently qualified and ask for their feedback. More often than not, they will give you invaluable advice and impressions that will make a significant impact on the way you work.

After a few minor adjustments to your image, role and technique, you will find that you soon progress into a comfortable and confident way of working with others, automatically adjusting your methods and style to individual needs.

Never allow complacency to creep in; always be aware of the need to reassess, adapt and respond to differing client requirements.

Protecting yourself

In this age of litigation and claims, it is important to ensure you have sufficient insurance cover as a professional aromatherapist.

If until now you have had student insurance, ask your insurance broker to change your policy to reflect your qualified status.

If you already have practitioner insurance for another discipline, ensure that the policy will also cover you for aromatherapy treatments.

Your college or aromatherapy organisation will be able to advise you of different tailor-made practitioner insurance schemes available. See also the Useful Addresses and Resource Guide.

Much of the following information originates from David Balen, the in-house Independent Financial Adviser of H and L Balen and Company, who specialise in providing insurance schemes for complementary therapists in the UK. There are different types of cover to choose from. The three most essential forms of cover include:

1. Public liability
This protects you if a member of the public is injured or put at risk whilst on your premises. Falling down the stairs or tripping over a rug are examples when public liability may be claimed. It may also include damage to their property if you are home visiting.

2. Medical malpractice
This covers you against harm inflicted on your client as a result of your treatment or advice if you have not acted with a reasonable degree of skill and care. An example might be a client claiming against you for using an essential oil that they were allergic to, resulting in serious skin sensitivity.

3. Professional indemnity
This covers you for loss claimed as a result of your conduct where injury has not occurred. An example of this might be if, as a consequence of your advice, a client decides to take a week of unpaid leave from work. His or her employer might be able to claim against you for loss of earnings that resulted.

There are many other forms of insurance cover that you may wish to consider. They include:

Product liability
Currently, if you give an essential oil blend you have used with your client as part of your treatment, you are covered by your malpractice insurance. However, if you plan to recommend or sell products such as formulas, blends or supplements to customers, you will require additional product insurance.

Therapy room contents
You can also be protected against loss or damage to the contents of your treatment room up to a certain value. This cover may also extend to your equipment when home visiting.

Property insurance
If you are working from home, your ordinary household insurance will not necessarily cover you for loss or damage to your couch, oils and other items. Consult with your insurance company at the earliest opportunity, as if you fail to disclose changes to your household arrangements, you may find that your ordinary household insurance is no longer valid.

Employers liability
This is a legal requirement for all employers. It covers you for injuries sustained by your employees. If you employ any person in your business, whether they be a cleaner, work experience assistant, receptionist or therapist, you must take out this cover and display the documentation on your premises.

Answering questions regarding insurance

Aromatherapy is such a safe therapy. Do I really need insurance?
It is a sign of the times that people are becoming increasingly litigious. This has little to do with whether aromatherapy is safe or not; claims may be made against you that have nothing directly to do with the therapy itself. Indeed, there are a few unscrupulous persons who make their living out of claiming off other people's insurance schemes!

What should I do if someone threatens to make a claim against me?
Firstly, do not panic, admit liability or mention your insurance company. Do not be tempted to enter into private negotiations for settlement. Deal with the threat swiftly, contact your insurer and pass on all correspondence to the insurance underwriters.

Do I require insurance if I am being employed as a therapist?
Employers should have all the necessary insurance to cover the actions of their employees, including Employers Liability. However, it is always wise to confirm who is legally liable for claims that might be made, as an action could be taken directly against you rather than via the employer. Unless you are specifically named on the employer's insurance policy, it is wise to have your own insurance.

Gaining authority to practise
Some areas have local byelaws that concern the practice of certain therapies, particularly those that involve massage. Approach the Trading

Standards department of your local county council before setting up in business to find out if there are any restrictions. A licence usually incurs an annual fee and inspection of your working premises. You may also be required to comply with Fire and Safety regulations. This advice applies equally if you plan to work from home.

In the UK, the law demands that you have your name and address visible somewhere at your place of work. Additionally, if you wish to display your name on a sign outside your premises (on a brass plaque for example), you will require permission from your local council.

Gaining in confidence

Confidence comes with practical application. There are no short cuts! If you find that you have few clients in the early stages, do not despair. Take this opportunity to:

● study further

● have aromatherapy treatments yourself

● practise blending

● continue treating family and friends

● smile and project a confident image to others

● use your network of support

● practise creative visualization; picture satisfied clients and a full appointment book!

The key to confidence is to believe in yourself and keep up with your practical skills. It is common to enter a 'slump' soon after qualifying; avoid the temptation to immerse yourself in misery and self-doubt!

As your confidence and expertise build, you will find that you develop your own individual style as a therapist as opposed to rigidly sticking to what you were taught in your course. Providing you do not deteriorate in technique or practise unethically or unsafely, this is usually a sign of your professional development.

LOCATING AND CREATING YOUR WORK ENVIRONMENT

Finding the ideal working solution

The previous chapter helped you consider the different working options together with their relative advantages and disadvantages. You need to decide which approaches will work best for you.

Many therapists combine part-time work with their aromatherapy practice in the early stages. This is because it takes time to build a client base; in the initial months your aromatherapy earnings are likely to be low. Having a part-time supplementary job can help ease the pressure as your client base expands and your experience grows. It can also provide a welcome respite from the intensity of working as a therapist.

If looking for part-time work to augment your income, try and find something that is related in some way to your chosen path. This will help keep you fresh, stimulated and extending your skills and knowledge. Such work might include:

- running adult education classes in aromatherapy

- working in a garden centre

- working in a health food shop that sells essential oils

- acting as receptionist in a complementary health clinic

- assisting in the day-to-day running of an essential oil company

- helping in the college where you trained.

Developing a therapeutic ambience

Once you have decided on how and where you wish to work, set about creating the ambience you feel most reflects your style of treatment. The ambience will vary according to your choice of location and the type of client you hope to attract. If you are planning to work from home or are leasing or buying specific premises, you will have the most freedom to create the 'perfect' clinic setting. It is also possible to create a therapeutic ambience in a rented clinic room or your client's home where you have less control.

Remember that above all, it is the client who needs to feel comfortable in the treatment space you have created. What make you feel relaxed and comfortable may not tally with your clients' expectations! Most clients will expect a treatment area to have a certain appearance, based on their previous experiences with their doctor and other practitioners. If you deviate too much from this image, you may find that clients are unable to relax and may not return for subsequent treatments.

In addition to your image as a therapist, there are other external factors that can help foster a therapeutic ambience that enhances your credibility and inspires confidence in your abilities:

- The careful use of colour, warmth and lighting can immediately help to put your client at ease, along with the impression of quiet, privacy and freedom from interruption.

- The availability of information regarding aromatherapy and the evidence of your training in the form of certificates or badges all helps to convey the message to your client that you are serious, professional and committed to standards.

- Your equipment and working area should be safe, clean and free of clutter.

Answering questions regarding ambience

How can I create a therapeutic ambience when I am home visiting?
Explain in advance to your client what a treatment entails. Encourage them to set aside an appointment time when they are going to have no distractions either during or immediately after the treatment. Ask them to ensure the room you will use will be warm for when you arrive. Ensure you allow time to set up your massage couch and arrange the room to maximise comfort, safety and relaxation.

Will music enhance the therapeutic ambience?
Many therapists use music in therapy. Sometimes it can be more for the benefit of the therapist than the client! If music is available, ask your client if they would like to listen to it. Tell them to feel able to ask for it to be stopped at any time. Music should enhance, not distract from the therapy. The Performing Rights Society provides a leaflet regarding using music on your premises. By law, if you intend to play copyright music for any purpose other than domestic use, you will require a PRS licence. See Useful Addresses and Resource Guide.

I do not have a separate changing room for my clients. How can I preserve their modesty?
This is a common scenario for therapists. Out of courtesy, you should consider leaving the room whilst they are dressing/undressing. At the very least, if you remain in the room, do not observe them whilst they are changing! Turning your back or occupying yourself with a task such as blending may be sufficient, depending on the client. Remember also to give clear instructions to your client as to how much clothing to remove for treatment to avoid anxiety and embarrassment.

Working with the medical profession

You may have a particular desire to work closely with the doctors and surgeries in your area. In your earlier networking period as a student, you will have developed an awareness for surgeries or individual doctors who are receptive to complementary therapies and who may be prepared to refer clients to you. Cultivate this relationship and ask clients who have gained significant relief from your care to keep their doctors informed of their progress.

Whenever a doctor or other practitioner refers a client to you, write them an initial courtesy letter of thanks followed by an update (with the client's permission) on his or her progress after a series of treatments.

Some doctor surgeries have spare consulting rooms that are rented out to practitioners of other disciplines. This can provide you with a remarkable opportunity to work closely with a medical team. To find out if this is a possibility for you, contact the practice manager or senior partner of the surgery concerned. If you are accepted to work within a medical setting, be prepared to work actively in educating both staff and clients as to the benefits and limitations of your work. You may also be asked to justify the use of certain oils or techniques; have quality literature sources and research references at hand.

PROMOTING YOUR SKILLS

Believing in yourself

Marketing is the art of promoting yourself and the services you offer. There are many different aspects, tools and techniques of marketing such as advertising and publicity but the goal is always the same: to attract clients who will want your services.

Self-confidence is your best marketing tool. You will make a positive impact if you believe in your work, gain enjoyment from it and can convey that impression to others. Always project a positive image – even if times are difficult and you are struggling to make ends meet. Do not think that pouring out your woes to other professionals will result in them referring clients to you out of pity! Projecting a positive image can be difficult at times and requires much courage and commitment but it always pays off.

Using effective marketing tools and techniques

When it comes to advertising and promotional literature, a good advertisement should be accurate, catchy, memorable and appropriately targeted.

The tried and tested **AIDA** principal is essential to follow when structuring your publicity:

A = attract *attention*

I = initiate *interest*

D = create *desire*

A = stimulate *action*

Bear in mind the additional points below:

● Keep your publicity concise, informative, in plain English and avoiding non-familiar jargon.

● Avoid flowery, ambiguous text that is difficult to read.

● Badly reproduced drawings or designs rarely make a good impression.

● Accuracy is important if you are to gain credibility and inspire confidence.

● Never deliberately mislead the public in the hope of attracting clients.

● If you are a member of an aromatherapy association, be sure not to breach their guidelines for advertising.

● There are firms that specialise in helping you promote your business.

Deciding where to advertise

This is an area fraught with pitfalls for the therapist. The precious budget you have set aside for advertising needs to be used wisely. It will be up to you to decide how and where best to promote your services. Common places to advertise are listed in Table 9 together with one advantage and disadvantage for each.

Keeping safe

If you are working from home, consider carefully whether to include your full address in your advertising. Are you prepared for people to 'call round' as they are passing by in order to make an appointment? Are you jeopardising your personal privacy and safety? Perhaps a pager or telephone number would be more appropriate to enable you to control visits and screen potential clients.

Table 9. Deciding where to advertise

Placement	Advantages	Disadvantages
local *Yellow Pages*	reliable, tried & tested	expensive
health magazines	appeal to interested audience	not targeted at local area
local papers	appeal locally	placement of advert often unsuitable
corner shop notices	appeal locally	dependent on the tone of other adverts
mail drop	can target specific areas	time-consuming to complete
natural health store/shop	appeal to interested persons	reliant on goodwill of shop owner

Cashing in on free advertising

1. *Let your clients sing your praises!* The most effective publicity tool is a satisfied client. Word of mouth is the best way to gain business. If your client expresses a wish to tell others, give them some leaflets or business cards to distribute amongst their friends and colleagues.

2. *Develop a good relationship with your local paper.* They may be willing to interview you or write up an account of your services free of charge.

3. *Offer to give free talks and demonstrations.* Local social and leisure clubs are often on the look out for interesting speakers and new topics.

Giving talks and demonstrations

This is an effective way of stimulating interest and generating potential clients. Not everyone feels comfortable with the thought of standing up in front of an audience and presenting themselves. Yet public speaking is a skill like any other – one that can be learnt. The key advice for giving a talk or demonstration is to prepare thoroughly for each session. Figure 10 lists 20 key pointers to successful public speaking.

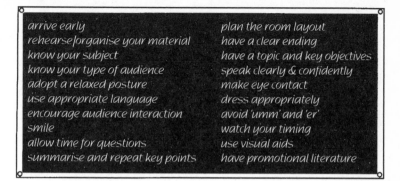

arrive early	plan the room layout
rehearse/organise your material	have a clear ending
know your subject	have a topic and key objectives
know your type of audience	speak clearly & confidently
adopt a relaxed posture	make eye contact
use appropriate language	dress appropriately
encourage audience interaction	avoid 'umm' and 'er'
smile	watch your timing
allow time for questions	use visual aids
summarise and repeat key points	have promotional literature

Fig.10. Tips for giving talks to the public.

MAINTAINING ACCURATE RECORDS

Fulfilling a legal obligation

The keeping of accurate and legible client records is a legal and professional requirement. This includes all client interactions including telephone calls. Every client that attends for treatment should be thoroughly consulted and all observations noted, with each intervention signed and dated. There are five main reasons for consulting and making client records:

1. aids choice of appropriate treatment approach

2. identifies cautions and contraindications

3. helps monitor progress and observe developing trends

4. helps protect you if a legal claim arises

5. indicates your interest and commitment to the client.

Your records should always be kept up to date and complete. Do not use Tippex or other correction fluids. Instead, cross through anything to be deleted in a way that it may still be read. The Medical Defence Union in the UK publishes a useful booklet concerning record keeping (see Further Reading and Useful Addresses and Resource Guide).

Avoiding judgmental observations

What you write in your client records is of vital importance. Under the

Access to Health Records Act 1990, clients have the right of access to any manually stored health records made since November 1991. The language you use in these records must therefore be unambiguous and accurate to the best of your knowledge.

For example, if your client during consultation confides to you that she is feeling depressed you might be tempted to record in your notes 'client is depressed'. Depending on the context, the words 'depressed' and 'depression' have different meanings. It would be better to include the client's own words 'I feel so depressed' to avoid an argument over the medical definition of depression in a court of law!

Do not use words or phrases that can be construed as judgmental or stereotypical. Your own personal reactions to an individual's personality or appearance may be unavoidable but they should not be recorded in the client's notes.

Some therapists ask their clients to read through their records at regular intervals and sign to confirm that they are a reliable account of what has taken place.

Storing records safely

To maintain client confidentiality, you should ensure that all notes and client records are stored appropriately, away from access by persons other than yourself. To avoid unprofessional practice, follow the advice below:

- Whilst you are in the clinic, ensure that other clients' notes are not lying on the desk in view of your present client.

- Never show a client's notes to another person without permission.

- If you wish to use a client's case history to present in class or for examination purposes, first ask the client's permission and omit the client's name and personal details to avoid identification.

- If you intend to store client details and records on computer, you will need to register with the Data Protection Agency. Your client has the right of access to these records as a result of the Data Protection Act 1998. For details regarding registration and obtaining a copy of the Act, refer to the Useful Addresses and Resource Guide.

SUMMARY

Now that you are qualified, the emphasis on preparedness and professionalism is even greater than before. It is always better to do something
correctly from the start than try and change when habits have set in.

- Establish clearly your image and role.
- Obtain all necessary insurance and authorisation to practise.
- Promote yourself positively.
- Seek out opportunities to tell others of your work.
- Strive always to create a therapeutic ambience.
- Keep accurate records.

The next chapter helps you cultivate a therapeutic relationship with your
clients.

CASE STUDIES

Jane joins forces with other professionals

Jane has decided to rent space in a multi-disciplinary clinic for one and
a half days a week in a prominent high street location. The clinic has a
good reputation in the area and a professional image. The rental rate is
high but Jane considers it a wise move and plans to extend the number
of days worked at the clinic within six months. She has negotiated a special start-up rate for the initial three months of her lease to help her get
established and has volunteered to give a talk and demonstration on aromatherapy to the receptionists, other practitioners and existing clinic
clientele.

Theresa begins at home

Upon qualification, Theresa held an aromatherapy party and invited
family, friends and hospice workers round to talk about her work and
show them her 'treatment room' based in the study of her home. At the
party, she gave each person a gift voucher for a sample treatment and
encouraged them to tell others about her work. In order to use the study
as a treatment room, she consulted the local authorities to find out if she
needed a licence to practise. Her local hospice has agreed for her to
attend for half a day per week initially to assess response and demand for
her treatments.

Mark makes a few changes

Having extended his existing practitioner insurance to cover his new qualification, Mark sent a letter to all his existing clients explaining his additional role as an aromatherapist. He put up leaflets and posters around the leisure centre and vaporised essential oils in the gym to stimulate interest. When he began giving aromatherapy treatments, he found that the clinical appearance of his treatment room inhibited some clients. He thus incorporated more pastel shades and installed a dimmer switch to modify the degree of lighting. He put up a curtain to hide technical equipment such as ultrasound and anatomical models when they were not required. He soon found that clients were able to relax deeply and gain the full benefits of an aromatherapy session.

THINKING IT THROUGH

1. Insurance brokers advise against displaying your certificates of professional indemnity or public liability in your working premises. Why do you think this advice is given?

2. Try and find non-judgmental words and phrases to replace the following:

   fat bossy weak unkempt dirty aggressive lazy unfit

3. It is important that the wording on your publicity material accurately reflects your image and role. What information have you included that conveys the work that you do?

8

Establishing Professional Relationships

Your training will have introduced you to the techniques and skills of effective client handling and communication. This chapter gives you key tips and reminders now that you are qualified and putting into practice all that you have learned. The art of keeping clients and fostering therapeutic relationships is as important as finding clients in the first place.

FOUNDING A THERAPEUTIC RELATIONSHIP

Assessing the needs of the client

There are basic and common needs that every client will share. These include physical, emotional and spiritual needs, a few of which are listed in Table 10.

The only sure-fire way of ascertaining the individual needs of the client is to actively **listen** and **observe**. Once you think you have gathered all the clues and grasped the message, be sure to verify it with the client. In this way, *together* you arrive at an agreed statement of needs and therefore purpose of treatment. These needs will evolve and change with progressive sessions; evaluate, listen and observe with each new session.

Table 10.   Basic client needs

Physical needs	emotional needs	spiritual needs
to be healed	to be heard	to be nourished
to be whole	to be accepted	to belong
to be soothed	to be loved	to find themselves
to be safe	to be reassured	to feel at peace

Encouraging a working partnership

In Chapter 1, the basic concepts of an holistic approach to health were outlined. One of the key underlying notions is that the individual is responsible for their own healing process, and that the therapist merely acts as a facilitator or catalyst to this end. Thus a truly holistic aromatherapy treatment programme is one in which the therapist and the client work *together* towards achieving better health and well-being.

Many clients accustomed to an allopathic approach to health will not be expecting such an holistic approach. They will be coming to you with the expectation that you will 'fix' their problem for them with a minimum of participation on their part. To encourage more client involvement:

● Actively listen to their story.

● Be interested in all aspects of their health and well-being.

● Ask for their response and feedback to the treatments.

● Involve them in your oil selection and treatment approach.

● Create a safe environment for them to focus on themselves.

● Create space for reflection and relaxation.

● Refer them to other professionals as needed.

Meeting the needs of the client

Having ascertained the needs and expectations of the client, you then need to consider the best course of action and decide if aromatherapy is suitable for that individual. There will be times when it is obvious that your client requires help from a different source. An example might be a client who has a need of medical assistance or specialised counselling. Do not bite off more than you can chew. Be honest and realistic with both yourself and your client and remember not to make claims or promises that what you do will bring relief.

Avoiding pedestals and unrealistic images

One of the most fulfilling aspects of your work as an aromatherapist is to participate in the transformation of clients with whom you work. Be it the relief of pain, the breaking of a pattern of insomnia or the processing of grief, you will gain an enormous amount of satisfaction from the work that you do. Pride and job satisfaction are positive and essential qualities. Remember to balance them with humility and deep respect for the people that you treat.

Grateful clients will frequently place you on a higher level than themselves. Pedestals are lonely, stressful and unstable places! Whilst they may be temporarily good for your ego and self-esteem, long-term they can harm the very therapeutic relationships you are trying so hard to build. If you feel your client has unacceptably high expectations of your capabilities, the easy response is to try and match it. The more difficult route is to explore the issue with your client and establish goals that are more realistic. Here are a few tips to avoid the stress of unrealistic expectations:

1. *Be human!* You are allowed to make mistakes, get ill and not know all the answers.

2. *Step down!* Keep the client as the priority. The moment you feel you are more important than the client, you have a pedestal problem.

3. *Let go!* Feel comfortable about referring clients to other practitioners. You will not always have the skills to treat every client that comes to you.

BUILDING TRUST AND RAPPORT

Fostering a trusting relationship

One of the most effective ways in which to build trust and rapport is to establish clear boundaries and ground rules with your client from the outset. In this way, there is no muddy area where your role is not distinct and your client will feel secure. The minimum boundaries you should establish at the beginning include:

● the duration of the session

● the fees

● the type of treatment

● the purpose of the treatment

● the number of planned treatments.

Both the fees and duration of the session are particularly important. Plan always to end your treatments on time. Do not feel that your client gains more benefit or respects you more if you run over time with each session. Once you have agreed a fee for your treatment, do not change it or waive it unless there are special circumstances.

Giving advice and recommendations

You will be asked on many occasions by your clients to give advice and personal opinions on matters relating to their health and well-being. This is a normal consequence of developing a trusting relationship. However, this is an area to tread with caution. It can be very hard to restrain from giving advice on a subject that you feel emotive about.

Only advise on subjects that are within your sphere of competence and expertise. This may include, for example, information on how to use essential oils at home or the selection of a suitable book on aromatherapy.

Common subjects that may not be within your sphere of competence include:

- nutritional supplements
- medication
- vaccinations
- weight loss programmes
- exercise regimes
- other complementary therapies.

If you do give advice, make it clear that the client is not obliged to follow it! Clients need to make an independent decision for themselves.

Remember also that if you are recommending, selling or passing on products to your clients, you will require product liability insurance.

RESPECTING INDIVIDUALITY

Practising a non-judgmental attitude

Great progress can be made when your client perceives that you are taking them seriously as an individual in an atmosphere of acceptance and unconditional positive regard. Sometimes this can be difficult if your client is seriously disfigured or has significantly different social or cultural circumstances from your own.

If you are giving advice regarding sensitive issues such as weight loss, stopping smoking or reducing alcohol intake, ensure that you are in no way conveying a judgmental attitude. If your client does not choose to follow this advice, it is not your place to scold or chide. You will need to respect their decision without annoyance or hint of selfrighteousness. If a client feels judged by you, this may lead to inhibition, distress and feelings of guilt.

Maintaining confidentiality

The previous chapter discussed ways to preserve confidentiality with regard to client records. Your client will also need to be reassured that you will not divulge information about them verbally to others without their prior permission. If you work with other practitioners in a clinic setting, avoid discussing shared clients unless it is in the context of planning appropriate care. You may find it difficult at times to maintain individual confidentiality when working with members of the same family; make sure you keep complete records of who said what and when to avoid breaches! The Medical Defence Union publishes a booklet concerning client confidentiality (see Further Reading and Useful Addresses and Resource Guide).

COMMUNICATING EFFECTIVELY

Using four senses of communication

It has been said that up to 70 per cent of communication takes place at a non-verbal level. An aromatherapy treatment is a powerful means of communication for several reasons. Taking full advantage of non-verbal opportunities to convey appropriate messages to your client will enhance your treatment.

Smelling

The aroma of your selected essential oil blend is a crucial part of your treatment. Allow your client the opportunity to deeply inhale its fragrance and let it make an impact on their psyche during the treatment itself. Do not confuse this aromatic encounter with bad breath, body odour, strong perfume or after-shave!

Touching

Your quality of touch is an integral part of the therapy whether it is the initial welcoming handshake or an aromatherapy massage itself. Ask yourself what you are communicating through your touch – support, acceptance and confidence or tension, impatience and boredom? Continuously assess the quality of your touch interaction with your client.

Seeing

During the initial welcome and consultation with your client, observation of body language and establishing eye contact is essential. However, don't overdo it! The eyes can convey reassurance, acceptance and confidence. What are your client's eyes telling you? Are they anxious, sad or fearful? During the treatment itself, eye contact is not always necessary as many clients find it helpful to close their eyes, relax and focus on the treatment.

Hearing

Listening to what your client is telling you is one of the arts of consultation. If you do not actively listen to your client, they will quickly perceive your disinterest. Additionally, outside noise such as telephones ringing, traffic and slamming doors can significantly disrupt a treatment session. Both what you say and how you say it has a deep impact on your client. Do not feel obliged to have all the answers. Avoid talking about yourself during the treatment. Remember who is the client and who is the therapist!

Communicating through silence

A treatment session provides the client with the opportunity to listen to their bodies and get in touch with their feelings. This is an important aspect of healing. In order to facilitate this process, try and minimise distraction and noise generated by yourself or others. This includes not initiating unnecessary conversation and working smoothly with confidence and awareness.

For some, part of the healing process involves the need to talk and express themselves. For others, chatting is a way of relieving nervous tension. This is appropriate when instigated by the client. Try and ensure that conversation remains focused and relevant to the treatment rather than serving to pass the time. Create the ambience that allows your client to feel comfortable with silence.

Remember that the aromas of the oils and the quality of your touch are already 'talking' to the client. Allow their impressions the chance to be 'heard'.

CREATING A SAFE ENVIRONMENT

Recognising the risks

To be safe is one of the basic needs and rights of any individual. With regard to the therapy environment, the issue of safety has several facets.

Table 11 outlines four main elements of safety together with risks and simple steps you can take to avoid their occurrence.

Protecting yourself

There will not always be the opportunity to screen the type of person you meet in therapy. There will be people attending for treatment who have complex unresolved issues within themselves that may make them

Table 11. Elements of safety

1. Environment

Risks	Avoiding Action
Faulty equipment	Check all equipment and electrical items regularly
Fire	Keep fire exit clear, know evacuation procedures
Unsafe surroundings	Ensure premises and furnishings are in good repair

2. Personal Possessions

Risks	Avoidinfg Action
Theft of belongings	Store items of value in a safe place
Damage to home furnishings	Care with preparing treatment area if home visiting
Spoilage of clothes/ furnishings	Attention to avoid spillage

3. Physical Health

Risks	Avoiding Action
Allergy	Consult thoroughly, patch test if necessary
Skin reactions	Use oils at correct dilution, evaluate sensitivity
Worsening of condition	Act within sphere of competence
Medical crises, e.g. fits, faints	Attend First Aid classes, keep First Aid box stocked

4. Emotional Health

Risks	Avoiding Action
Embarrassment	Maintain modesty and privacy
Guilt	Create a non-judgmental rapport
Breach of confidentiality	Store records carefully, discuss issue with client
Fear of breaking down	Convey acceptance, establish a support system

angry, threatening or prone to violence. If you are working from home, your vulnerability may be increased. You may wish to ensure that there is always another person in the home when you meet a client for the first time. When home visiting, make an attempt to assess the client's motivation for treatment before the initial visit. If you feel that a client in any way compromises your safety, do not feel obliged to continue treating them.

Avoiding sexual exploitation

Some people find it hard to separate sensuality from sexuality. Thus they may develop a sexual response to your touch and/or essential oil choice. This rarely happens if you have been able to project a professional image and have clearly established boundaries and ground rules. In the event of such a response, it is important to remain calm, professional and non-judgmental. It may be a transient event that in no way affects the treatment process. However, if the response persists and is becoming intrusive to your work, a suggestion is that you inform your client that the treatment has come to an end and that you will return once they are clothed. Leave the room and give them time to compose themselves. You may then wish to discuss the event openly with the client and re-clarify your role as a therapist.

Maintaining your privacy

Building a rapport with clients is an essential part of their healing process. The balance between a healthy rapport and an unhealthy one is very delicate. There is a real risk of becoming over-involved with your client and divulging too much about your personal life. Remember that as a therapist, you do not have to be 'public property'; there may remain areas of your life that are private. This can be quite difficult to preserve with certain clients who ask you questions about your personal life and circumstances. How much information you choose to divulge is up to you and not for the client to decide.

SUMMARY

The therapeutic relationship you build with each client has a direct impact upon the course and outcome of the treatment. This chapter has encouraged you to:

● consider the needs of the client

- establish a working partnership

- build an atmosphere of rapport and trust

- communicate effectively on all levels

- maintain a safe therapeutic environment.

The next chapter helps you avoid the common pitfalls of being a therapist.

CASE STUDIES

Jane initially struggles with confidence
The first few months of working as an aromatherapist were difficult for Jane. She felt daunted by the prospect of treating 'real, live, paying' clients and consequently found herself projecting an overly tense and serious image. She was particularly afraid that her clients would lose confidence if she had to use her reference books. Having other practitioners at hand in the clinic to give advice and support was invaluable. She gradually developed warmer, more trusting relationships with her clients and felt less inhibited about checking oil choices.

Theresa starts to clarify her role
In the initial few months, Theresa found it difficult to step into the role of a therapist when family and friends came for treatment. Consequently she felt frustrated by the informality and felt she was not giving them the best of her care despite spending extra time and effort. She thus made a conscious decision to clarify her role with people wanting treatment. In turn, they came to respect her boundaries and adopted the role of clients rather than friends. By making appointments and keeping to the time allocated, together they worked out a secure therapeutic relationship that existed outside their friendship.

Mark learns from his clients
Having modified his treatment room to take into account the needs of his clients, Mark soon discovered there were more changes to be made. He found that using essential oils with his work allowed him to adopt a softer, more sensitive role than his normally strong and technical role as a sports therapist. He now listens more to the emotional needs of each client and responds accordingly.

THINKING IT THROUGH

1. Client confidentiality and trust are emphasised as essential aspects of a client/therapist relationship. On what occasions might there be legitimate cause for breaching them without the consent of the client?

2. How might you respond to a satisfied client who asks you to make an essential oil blend and give advice concerning a member of their family?

3. Consider how you might handle a client who consistently makes and breaks appointments, arrives late and yet tells you how important your treatments are for their health and well-being.

9

Avoiding the Pitfalls

Having taken so much time and care to plan your aromatherapy career, it is important to ensure it is long lasting and that your skills and job satisfaction increase as time goes by. This chapter helps you to avoid common mistakes that therapists of all disciplines encounter and gives you tips for developing your own personal therapist survival plan.

COMBINING CARING WITH EARNING

Recognising the dilemma

If you talk with other therapists of caring disciplines, you will commonly find that the issue of charging and accepting money for treatments is an uncomfortable one. As already discussed in Chapter 2, many carers find it hard to place a price on what they do and frequently under-charge. Here are three reminders on how to balance giving with receiving:

1. Develop a healthy attitude towards money.

2. Acknowledge your true value.

3. Try and separate your emotions from the act of receiving money.

If you are truly unable to reconcile your work with accepting payment, one possible solution is to make arrangements so that someone else charges and accepts payment on your behalf. This might be a partner if you are working from home or the receptionist if you are working in a clinic. Whatever solution you find most comfortable, ensure that you neither under-charge nor undervalue your skills.

Taking time out

A common misconception of the self-employed is that you are unable to take breaks or holidays for fear of losing clients and valuable income. With careful planning and time management, taking regular breaks should become an essential perk and part of your freedom as a self-employed person with no threat to your existing client base or financial state. A timely break away can refresh, recharge, give you an added perspective on your skills, and your clients will gain benefit from your energy and well-being. You are not indispensable! If you give your clients advance notice that you will be away, you will find that your planned holiday will bring you immense benefit and your clients will still be there when you return.

Valuing family and friends

There is a risk of becoming so immersed in your clients' problems that you lose sight of the needs of family and friends. This is not a conscious process and it may be that you are the last person to notice! Finding the balance between home and work is an ever-challenging task. If you feel that you are skipping social engagements, denying yourself and missing out on quality time with family and friends, it is likely that your priorities have become distorted. Act quickly and take steps to redress the balance.

Learning to say 'no'

Assertiveness is a skill that many therapists are afraid of using. By not being able to say 'no' and failing to establish clear boundaries, therapists of all disciplines run the risk of over-committing and overstretching themselves. Driven by the desire to please and the fear of rejection, a lack of assertiveness leaves the door open to abuse of many sorts. Typical examples where assertiveness skills may be needed include:

● clients telephoning you at home

● demands for treatment outside your normal working hours

● people who try and involve you directly in their problems

● clients who use emotional manipulation to their own gain.

Being assertive is a positive quality; it improves your self-confidence and conveys clear messages to others. If you find it difficult to say no, you may wish to start by practising self-assertion in a controlled and safe environment. You may find there are classes in assertiveness being conducted in your area.

AVOIDING BURN OUT

Recognising the signs

The phenomenon of burnout is particularly common amongst people working within the caring professions. The demands of clients and financial pressures can be extremely exhausting and seemingly relentless at times. It is important not to over-stretch yourself on any level. Common factors contributing to burnout include:

- fear of rejection
- fear of failure
- poor time management
- low self-esteem
- perfectionism
- unrealistic expectations
- financial insecurity
- lack of assertiveness
- always trying to please
- becoming over-involved emotionally
- physical overload.

Table 12 includes different behavioural, emotional and physical signs of burnout. On their own, these general signs are not indicative of burnout, but when a group of them exist, there is a possibility that you may be at risk. If you allow yourself to become chronically over-stressed, you have stopped listening to your body and are on the road to ill health.

Taking practical steps

If you identify with a number of the signs in Table 12, ask yourself what you would advise a client to do in a similar position, and then follow your own advice! It is common to be so busy caring for others that you neglect your own needs. In order to give truly to others, you need also to give to yourself.

Here are fifteen ways to avoid burnout and develop a personal survival plan:

1. Take regular time out.
2. Pay attention to exercise and diet.

Table 12. Signs of burnout

low self-esteem	on 'automatic pilot'
ignoring personal needs	inattention to diet
feeling helpless	unable to make decisions
panic attacks	fatigue
hyperventilation	decline in performance
feelings of resentment	making mistakes
poor judgment	lapses in concentration
sense of hopelessness	feelings of guilt
lack of job satisfaction	behavioural changes
altered sleeping habits	mood changes
poor personal	increase in common
relationships	ailments
increase in smoking	desire to run away
increase in alcohol	unable to step out of
consumption	therapist's role

3. Cultivate healthy relationships.

4. Have a social life.

5. Guard your private life.

6. Avoid pedestals and unrealistic expectations.

7. Develop a hobby.

8. Have treatments from other therapists.

9. Deal with your own personal issues as they arise.

10. Avoid over-stretching.

11. Learn to say 'no'; establish boundaries.

12. Keep a healthy self-esteem.

13. Mentally separate work and home.

14. Learn to detach emotionally from your clients.

15. Use your network of support.

Combining sensitivity with detachedness

As a therapist, being able to stand back and act as a catalyst to healing is far more effective than joining with the client and trying to solve their problems. To be objective and detached does not imply that you do not care. On the contrary, it reflects your deep commitment and respect for your clients.

Some therapists are particularly sensitive to the energy, moods and physical state of other people. They are able to sense intimately the client's needs and problems and subsequently find it difficult to extricate themselves at the end of the treatment without feeling affected energetically, emotionally or physically.

If you identify with this sensitivity, you will need to find your own way of protecting yourself against becoming drained or adversely affected by each client you treat. Many therapists use meditation, imagery and creative visualization to replenish lost energy and protect themselves between clients, These techniques are simple to learn and apply. If your college has not already given you advice regarding sensitivity, ask other therapists in your support network what steps or techniques they use.

MAKING A DISTINCTION BETWEEN WORK AND HOME

Changing roles

Another pitfall of being a therapist is the risk of remaining in 'therapist mode' once you finish work and your role has changed. This can lead to increased stresses in your personal relationships. To avoid this, develop your own technique and routine of making the transition. It may include:

- having a half hour on your own

- taking a bath or shower

- changing into fresh clothing

- meditating

- walking the dog

- taking active exercise.

Setting aside quality time

In order to remain fresh and avoid burnout, incorporate quality time out with family and friends. To come home each day exhausted and spend the evening with family in a semi-awake state is not quality time! Plan in advance and make a firm mental commitment to create opportunities for fun, relationships and personal enjoyment.

USING ESSENTIAL OILS SAFELY

Considering toxicity

In your aromatherapy studies, you will have learnt the risks of inappropriate essential oil use, with particular reference to your client. Be aware that as a therapist using essential oils on a regular basis, you are more at risk from possible adverse effects than clients who attend at different intervals. During a single clinic day, you are exposing yourself to a veritable 'cocktail' of different essential oil blends via both skin absorption and inhalation.

Although essential oils are remarkable tools with limited risk when used appropriately, over-use of any substance is potentially hazardous. The long-term risk to aromatherapists from continuous essential oil use is as yet unknown. It is therefore wise always to exercise caution. Non-specific symptoms that may signal over-use include:

● increase in tiredness

● headaches

● nausea

● change in menstrual cycle

● lack of concentration

● increase in common ailments.

Specific symptoms in direct response to using certain oils include:

(a) irritation

(b) rashes

(c) eczema/dermatitis.

Minimising the risks

Here are ten tips for all people using essential oils on a regular basis:

1. Work in a well-ventilated area.

2. Avoid unnecessary contact with undiluted essential oils.

3. Wear gloves to mop up spillages.

4. Vary the essential oils you use.

5. Have at least one day per week when essential oils are not used.

6. Keep well hydrated.

7. Wash your hands regularly.

8. Take regular breaks throughout the day.

9. Irrespective of your client's needs, do not use essential oils that you have identified as personally sensitising.

10. Avoid the continual use of the same essential oil over long periods of time.

Staying healthy

Remember to practise what you preach! Adopt a moderate and healthy lifestyle wherever possible. Eat well, breathe fresh air, take exercise, laugh and enjoy life. Cultivate healthy relationships with others and do not ignore your own health problems.

SUMMARY

This practical chapter will have helped you to:

- receive appropriate financial gain for your work

- recognise the warning signs of burnout

- plan and take action to keep fresh and effective

- place value on yourself and your family

- avoid putting your own health at risk in the course of helping others.

The next chapter encourages you to continue with your professional development and maintain your effectiveness as a therapist.

CASE STUDIES

Jane's energy takes a nosedive

After almost a year, Jane's aromatherapy practice is booming. She has increased her clinic time to four full days per week and she visits immobile clients in their own homes. The pressure to earn a living and her sense of responsibility to her clients is starting to take a toll. She is finding that she spends much of her home time worrying about clients and thinking about further ways in which to help them. She has not taken a holiday since she began her aromatherapy studies and despite feeling drained and stressed emotionally, is reluctant to take a break for fear of 'letting her clients down'.

Theresa is increasingly out of pocket

Theresa continues to have difficulties juggling work and home commitments. Her particular problem concerns charging people at home for the treatments she gives. Additionally, her family feels that their home-life and privacy is intruded when she treats clients at weekends and evenings. Her voluntary work at the hospice has expanded following a positive response and she feels guilty about asking the hospice to help with her expenses. Despite the satisfaction of helping others with aromatherapy, Theresa is starting to realise that her services are being used rather than valued.

Mark deals with isolation

Mark is making great strides combining his aromatherapy practice with his other skills. He has a well-organised fee structure and keeps weekends free for his recreational activities. He has received much publicity in the local press and has been asked to lecture at a few sports conferences. However, as a male aromatherapist in the field of sports medicine, he has found very few people locally with whom to compare experiences. A friend suggests he may find others working in a similar field through the Internet. After several postings to various lists and discussion groups, he makes contacts with others around the world who are involved in similar activities. His sense of isolation starts to lessen.

THINKING IT THROUGH

1. You may remember that Jane experienced similar problems of over-commitment as a student. What steps might she take now as a professional aromatherapist to avoid impending burnout?

2. How might 'Theresa be able to detach her feelings from receiving adequate payment for her services and appease her family? Does her attitude convey messages regarding her own self-esteem?

3. Developing a personalised therapist survival plan can help you avoid the risks of burnout and remain an efficient and professional therapist. Which areas have you personally identified as needing attention and action?

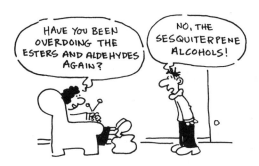

10

Consolidating Your Skills

A challenging aspect of your role as a therapist is the fact that you never stop learning. Therapists are perpetual students! The opportunities to augment your knowledge, develop additional skills and grow in your professional life abound. This chapter seeks to suggest ways to remain fresh, current and enthusiastic about your work.

KEEPING UP WITH NEW DEVELOPMENTS

Staying abreast

Aromatherapy is described by many as an evolutionary therapy that has reached the stage of adolescence; a phase of turbulence, change, transformation, challenge and opportunity. Times move fast; aromatherapy in particular has witnessed immense change. Over the past twenty years, aromatherapy has moved from being an unknown therapy to one of the most popular forms of complementary medicine in the UK.

In times such as these, it is easy to get left behind and lose touch with the evolution of the therapy as a whole. It is crucial to remain current if you wish to maintain a long-term career. Aromatherapy associations, colleges and training standards have also been challenged to keep pace with these changes. It is therefore likely that such standards will be subject to frequent review and updating for the foreseeable future. These changes may affect your eligibility to remain a member of your aromatherapy association. If you do not stay current with developments, you may lose your membership rights. Here are five tips for staying current:

1. Subscribe to aromatherapy journals (see Useful Addresses and Resource Guide).

2. Keep in touch with your college and your aromatherapy associates.

3. Meet fellow aromatherapists on a regular basis.

4. Attend aromatherapy workshops, seminars and conferences.

5. Keep records of all courses/workshops attended to demonstrate your commitment to professional development.

Keeping current with the health industry

It is also wise to keep your eyes on changes and emerging trends within the health industry as a whole. These aspects of the wider picture may positively or negatively affect your career opportunities.

An example of positive developments was the publication in October 1997 of *Integrated Healthcare: a Way Forward for the Next Five Years*. This report by the Foundation of Integrated Medicine made many proposals regarding the future of both orthodox and complementary medicine, including suggestions concerning training, research and self-regulation of therapies.

An example of possibly negative developments that may influence your career is the continuing debate as to whether herbal products and essential oils should be classed as medicines and thus subject to regulations regarding licensing and dispensation. Changes within the European Union may have direct implications for the future of complementary therapies in the United Kingdom. It is important, therefore, to keep informed of changes and give support wherever necessary to uphold and protect the therapy profession.

To stay current with the general climate of natural health care:

● Subscribe to natural health journals (see Useful Addresses and Resource Guide).

● Maintain regular contact with professionals of other disciplines.

● Attend debates, conferences and workshops on different aspects of complementary medicine.

UPDATING YOUR KNOWLEDGE

Keeping fresh

Your original level of training provided you with a foundation to your therapy and yet only signals the beginning of your studies. The sense of discovery and deep respect for the intricacy of the human body and the sheer diversity of clients that you treat will ensure that you keep learning and growing as a therapist.

By extending your skills and embarking on further studies, you are enriching and nourishing yourself as well as your clients. Take regular time out to study. It is never wasted and keeps your interest and experience alive and fresh.

Studying alone

With the diversity of literature written about aromatherapy, there will never be a shortage of books to read to further your understanding and concepts. Remember to read selectively, with an open mind, and be prepared to filter what you read. Incorporate your new learning only after critical evaluation and careful consideration.

Having undergone aromatherapy training that has focused upon a particular facet of the therapy, you will recognise that no single course is entirely complete; it usually reflects the understanding and views of that particular college. You may wish to get a broader grasp of the therapy as a whole by studying with different teachers. Correspondence courses offer opportunities to study and gain new insights without having to take further time off work.

Using the Internet

If you have access to the Internet, there are many discussion groups and sites relating to aromatherapy and other aspects of natural medicine. This greatly widens your understanding and appreciation of the therapy as a whole and enables you to correspond with those who share your interests around the world. Using one of the many built-in search engines of your web browser, thousands of sites may be found by typing 'aromatherapy' or 'essential oil'.

Studying with others

It is particularly refreshing to take time out to participate in courses attended by other aromatherapists. Information about such postgraduate events may be found by contacting:

- your college

- aromatherapy associations

- essential oil companies

- journals of aromatherapy and natural healthcare.

At such events you are likely to meet aromatherapists of varying specialties and experience with whom you can share and discuss your work.

Many therapists attending postgraduate events state that the coffee and lunch breaks are as great a learning opportunity as the lectures themselves!

Continuing your studies

You may find that your aromatherapy training serves as a launch pad for the study of other therapies and professions. As the basic training incorporates so many different subjects, the desire for further study may lead you into a related dimension of care. Beware, however, of the risk of being 'a jack of all trades and master of none'. If you do embark on further training, ensure it is undertaken in a thorough manner and give yourself time to assimilate your learning before moving onto a new therapy or subject. Related therapies and professions are listed in Table 13.

Table 13. Related therapies and professions

Herbal medicine	Horticulture
Reflexology	Osteopathy
Cranio-sacral therapy	Counselling
Nutrition	Acupuncture
Shiatsu	Crystal healing
Therapeutic Touch	Healing
Nursing	Sports therapy
Perfumery and cosmetic sciences	

EXTENDING YOUR SKILLS

Considering teaching aromatherapy

Experienced aromatherapists often combine their clinical practice with teaching others. This can create a related and fulfilling balance to the intensity of working in a clinic. Opportunities for teaching aromatherapy arise in different ways:

- adult education classes

- private tuition teaching within an established college

- working with doctors and medical students

- providing information on essential oils, their use and safety to sales staff.

To contribute effectively as an aromatherapy teacher, you will require an in-depth knowledge of your subject plus significant experience of its practical application. It is not something that is recommended if you are recently qualified. Usually a minimum of two years experience in practice is required for aromatherapy tutors in a college setting.

Learning how to teach

Effective teaching is a skill that may be acquired and developed through life experience or formal training. It is highly recommended that you embark upon some form of teacher training to enhance your communication and teaching ability; an appropriate qualification in the UK might be the City and Guilds 7307 Further and Adult Education Teachers Certificate. You will find books on adult education and details of such courses from your local library. Table 14 lists some common attributes of a teacher.

Table 14.   Common teacher attributes

time management	authority	clarity
preparation	interest	experience
sense of humour	patience	logic
method	enthusiasm	listening skills
management skills	flexibility	vocal projection
knowledge of subject	expertise in use of learning aids	communication skills
confidence	respect	commitment

EMBARKING ON RESEARCH

Understanding why research is important

In recent years there has been an increased demand upon all working within the health professions to justify the work they do in relation to:

- efficacy
- public safety
- time and cost-effectiveness.

This demand applies equally to therapists working within the alternative and complementary medicine sector. One inescapable fact is that if a therapy is to gain in recognition and become a respected part of integrated medicine, it will have to demonstrate unequivocally that it is safe, effective and affordable.

Many therapists see little relevance for research; you witness enormous benefit to clients on a daily basis and are therefore already confident that your therapy is safe, effective and affordable. So why bother to prove it?

Additionally, you may feel overawed by the jargon and unfamiliar methodologies associated with research and have negative memories from statistics lessons at school! Despite the negative images and popular misconceptions, there are positive advantages for the therapist involved in research:

1. It improves your practice.

2. It furthers your knowledge.

3. It adds credibility to your field.

4. It teaches you how to assess critically and objectively.

Some practical disadvantages of research include:

1. It may need significant funding.

2. It generally involves considerable time.

3. It may not confirm your initial expectations.

4. It may result in more questions than answers.

Doing your own research

In its simplest form, research relates to any endeavour to discover facts by careful study and systematic investigation. Thus research need not be on a grand scale. Examples of research that involves little time and expense in your own practice might be to:

● calculate the average age of your clients

● ascertain if seasonal changes appear to affect the number of clients making appointments.

The information you glean might be then put to good use when planning holidays or to help you organise an advertising campaign.

Objectively analysing your practice on a regular basis is a healthy form of research and professional development. It involves stepping off the treadmill long enough to stand back and assess aspects of your practice.

Appreciating the value of case studies
You may find that you are receiving great response to your treatments from clients with particular conditions. Your interest might lead you to investigate further the aspects of your treatment that most influence these clients. Gathering related case studies is an important baseline for research and may serve to launch a more formal study.

Working with others
If you decide to embark upon a more comprehensive research project, there are three golden rules:

1. Choose a topic that interests you.

2. Involve the expertise of others.

3. Have patience and sticking power.

The following section gives you brief advice regarding how to go about instigating a larger-scale research project.

Selecting a research topic
The topic you choose to research must be both interesting and relevant to your work otherwise you will run out of stamina before its completion! Additionally, you will need to conduct your own primary research in the form of literature searches to ascertain if anyone else has already studied what you are trying to do; there is little point in reinventing the wheel! By examining the research of others, you will also gain an idea of how to approach your study based upon their methods and results.

Ensure that your topic is specific and offers means of investigation using standard methods of measurement that can be reliably reproduced by others.

Preparing a research proposal
Having decided upon a topic and conducted a comprehensive literature review, the next step is to make a research proposal. This is a detailed written plan of the research you are intending to conduct. A proposal:

- helps you clarify the key points of the project
- communicates these points to others you wish to be involved
- is needed for obtaining support and funding.

A proposal is rarely more than one page long and covers all the main points of your planned research. Thus it needs to be concise and include:

1. title

2. abstract summary

3. literature review

4. methods and plan of investigation

5. budget and proposed time-frame for completion

6. evidence that you are a suitable person to conduct the research that you are proposing.

Gaining expert advice

The most important aspect about research is that it is done correctly; there have been numerous studies conducted by people who did not receive adequate advice and support regarding research design and implementation. The results, no matter how spectacular, do not carry weight in the light of scientific scrutiny if the methodology, design or analyses are flawed. This can be extremely discouraging for researchers who have spent a great deal of time and commitment on their study only to find that it is not accepted by the wider scientific community.

A simple way to avoid this outcome is to involve others whose daily work involves research design and implementation. They have the necessary professional expertise and resources that you require. If you have drawn up a clear research proposal, are able to demonstrate your commitment and have plans to publish your findings, it is likely that you will find the necessary people to give you guidance and support. Professionals you may need to involve include clinicians, scientists and research designers, plus the medical ethics committee attached to your local health authority.

Universities, colleges and establishments that already publish research in related subjects are more likely to be interested in your proposal. See the Useful Addresses and Resource Guide for possible contacts, sponsors and recommended reading concerning research.

Seeking sponsorship

There are establishments that are interested in offering support, advice and sponsorship to people with good research proposals. Your application may be one of many competing for a fixed sum of sponsorship; make sure yours is the one they select! Your college and aromatherapy association may have information regarding sponsors particularly interested in aromatherapy. Remember that sponsorship may also come from local sources, such as essential oil suppliers and local businesses. They are more likely to agree to sponsorship if you plan to acknowledge their contributions when the findings are published.

Staying focused

Once you have gained the resources and support to conduct your research, expect times when you wonder why you ever started! The seemingly interminable process of gathering data and making sense of it can challenge even the most experienced researcher. However, following a research project through to its completion, seeing it published and having the opportunity thereby to influence professional practice is an enormously rewarding experience. Remember the third golden rule – Have patience and sticking power!

SUMMARY

Stagnation is a condition that can adversely affect your future prospects and job satisfaction. It is thus important to advance your knowledge and skills on a regular basis. This chapter has encouraged you to:

- stay fresh and interested in what you do

- keep current with developments in your therapy and in healthcare as a whole

- extend your skills and consider further training

- consider research a useful and necessary aspect of your professional development.

The following and final chapter helps you to evaluate your progress and safeguard the future.

CASE STUDIES

Jane furthers her studies

Jane's commitment to her clients is reflected in the desire to keep current and develop new skills. She has found that she needs to plan carefully if she wants to attend postgraduate classes and seminars, and that the time, money and effort is well rewarded. Her current particular observation is that aromatherapy appears to work effectively for pain control. Her local doctor who regularly refers clients for aromatherapy encourages her to conduct a small pilot study with some of his clients who have arthritic pain. Unsure of how to embark upon such a project, she goes to her local library for a book on basic research skills to familiarise herself with standard methods before taking matters further.

Theresa branches out

Throughout her life, Theresa has been fascinated by the subtle concepts of health and healing. Her aromatherapy experiences have rekindled this interest. As a result, she has undertaken a course in healing and crystal therapy and has recently enrolled on a counselling course. She is gaining great fulfillment from helping in a gentle yet effective way, and her quiet, mature approach seems to instil confidence in others.

Mark finds his expertise is in demand

Mark's initial quest to augment his professional skills has not ended with his aromatherapy qualification; he continues to keep himself informed of changes in the professions he represents and the opportunities for further study. Through the Internet and his article contributions in professional journals, he has attracted international interest and is now starting to lecture and share his skills further afield. Additionally, he has been instrumental in incorporating basic aromatherapy training into the curriculum of some colleges of sports medicine.

THINKING IT THROUGH

1. There is an argument that a successful and full-time therapist will not have the time to undertake postgraduate training and that his or her learning is enhanced sufficiently through practical experience. What are your opinions?

2. One argument for not undertaking research into complementary therapies is that it goes against holistic principles. Another is that therapy effectiveness is impossible to measure using standard research methods. Do you agree?

3. How might you be able to begin incorporating aspects of analysis and research into your practice? Think of simple as well as more formal studies.

11

Reaping the Rewards

This last chapter combines reflection with forward thinking. The re-evaluation of primary goals and the setting of new targets are part of your ongoing travels in the therapy field. Numerous opportunities for growth and expansion will present themselves. It is time to consolidate as well as advance further along your chosen path.

ASSESSING PERSONAL AND FINANCIAL GAIN

Recognising growth and achievement

At regular intervals it is helpful to step back and reflect upon your accomplishments on both a personal and professional level. For example, what impact has your decision to become an aromatherapist had upon your life? Sometimes this form of reflection can be difficult to conduct alone as it needs a degree of objectivity. You may wish to ask family, friends or colleagues their opinions regarding your personal growth and achievements. They may provide insights that you have overlooked.

People have different ways of measuring success and failure. Financial gain is not always the most important test. All learning experiences have their share of positive and negative aspects.

Ask yourself . . .

1. If you have not become as wealthy as you had hoped, yet have grown in confidence and self-esteem, does this mean you have failed?

2. If having completed your training and attempted to make a career of aromatherapy, you decide to follow a completely different path, does this mean you have wasted your time?

3. If your success as an aromatherapist has been at the expense of a broken home life, does this mean you are fulfilled?

When you do reflect upon your achievement and growth, be honest, realistic and not overly self-critical. Acknowledge your efforts and accomplishments as well as the areas that did not meet your expectations.

Reflecting upon original aims and objectives

As a practical exercise, you may wish to consider your original aims and objectives for becoming an aromatherapist. In Chapters 1 and 2 you were encouraged to identify these together with your motives. Do you feel that you have met your targets? If you have, you will feel a deserved degree of self-satisfaction and accomplishment and will be ready to set new aims and objectives.

If you have not met your original aims and objectives, consider why this might be:

● Were your initial aims clearly defined?

● Were they realistic?

● Did you formulate a suitable plan to achieve them?

● Did you lose sight of them along the way?

● Did circumstances change?

● Did you change direction and follow different goals?

● Is it too soon to make an assessment?

Making changes

One of the purposes of self-assessment is to identify changes that need to be made in order to fulfil your original aims or to follow new ones. Drawing up an action plan is a positive and constructive task that clearly points you in the right direction.

An action plan is particularly useful if you have highlighted problems in your work or home life as it challenges you to deal with issues in an objective way. Looking upon your problems as challenges to overcome can help you deal with them effectively. Writing an action plan clarifies your thoughts and transforms them into workable ideas. You will gain most benefit if you can be specific about the changes you want to make.

Creating an action plan
An action plan consists of at least four parts:

1. identification of the area that requires change, the *challenge*

2. identification of your goal, the *expected outcome*

3. course of *action* to be taken

4. a realistic time-span for *review*.

Table 15 gives an example of a typical action plan.

Table 15. A typical action plan

Challenge	Tendency to run over time with clients
Expected outcome	Improved time management
Action to be taken	Place clock in a more visible place in treatment room
	Ensure clients are clear regarding appointment times and duration
	Avoid introducing new topics of conversation at the end of a session
	Use more verbal and non-verbal cues that the session is completed
Time for review	3 months = 1/10/XX Comments

Using financial gain wisely

Financial gain is not a guarantee of happiness but it can buy you time and the opportunity to do what you want to do. This degree of control and freedom to act in the way that you want is one of the main motives for earning money in the first place! Therefore, when circumstances and finances are favourable, take the opportunity to fulfil your aims.

Draw up a list of desires that require financial input for their fulfilment and then work towards their reality. Be it small or large, whatever is on your list of desires is important to you. Being able to fulfil each desire over a period of time will impart a great sense of achievement.

Thinking of the future
If you are self-employed, you may wish to consider your future financial

stability and take steps to ensure that you have adequate resources in case of illness, disability and when you retire. This may be in the form of investments or choosing one of the numerous private insurance and pension plans on offer to the self-employed. Financial advisers, banks and building societies offer advice regarding planning for your future. Shop around and seek expert advice to ensure you use your money wisely.

DEALING WITH SUCCESS

Combining pride and humility

One of the greatest joys and rewards of aromatherapy is to witness how a treatment can transform and empower. This creates an immense sense of well-being for both you and grateful clients. It is healthy to be proud of your achievements in becoming an aromatherapist. You have worked hard and are now reaping the rewards of good practice. Your confidence and self-esteem are important to your success.

Putting the client first

In the flush of success, however, pride has a tendency to run away with itself! When your ego gets in the way of your work, you will find that your long-term prospects of serving others are in jeopardy. To prevent this happening, always remember that it is the client who is the priority. It is an enormous privilege to work with those who allow you to question, probe and examine their innermost selves in such an intimate way. This calls for immense respect for the individual and true humility when working with others.

If you always keep the client as your priority, you will retain a balanced impression of your success whilst guarding your pride and preserving your self-esteem.

Being wary of the egos of others

In all walks of life you will come across highly experienced and charismatic people who attract a wide following of those eager to emulate them. In extreme cases, these people may become like gurus. The aromatherapy profession around the world has its share of people who may be subtly using the profession to attract attention and enact their own power game rather than purely acting for the benefit of the therapy. Whilst it may be extremely enriching to study with and learn from these people, ensure your experience is wide enough to be able to form your own opinions and develop your own independent ideas and flair.

Keeping your feet on the ground

You will have discovered that aromatherapy incorporates a broad spectrum of theories and practical applications. This adds to its versatility and attraction. At one extreme, you will find applications to clinical science with its emphasis on chemistry and bioactivity while the other extreme encompasses the subtle and intangible aspects of the energetic applications of essential oils. It is likely that you will be more comfortable and accepting of one particular pole and develop more skills in that direction. Bear in mind that in order to be balanced, you need to have at the very least a basic understanding and acceptance of all other aspects. To have your feet stuck in the cement of science or your head in the clouds of ethereal bliss both represent imbalances that need to be addressed. Figure 11 illustrates the necessary balance between the different aspects of aromatherapy.

REPRESENTING YOUR THERAPY

Reflecting the profession

Your work as a therapist is not just a matter between you and your clients; the image you project and your conduct carry wider messages regarding the profession you represent. Bear in mind that you are a spokesperson for your therapy every time you step into your therapist's role. Do nothing to bring your profession into disrepute. Your profession will expect you to convey:

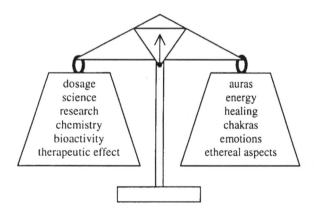

Fig. 11 Getting the balance right.

- integrity

- respect for others

- professionalism

- good conduct

- safe practice

- compliance with regulations

- honesty

- competence.

Every association has a professional code of conduct and ethics; ensure you have read through and comply with those of the associations to which you belong.

Opening the doors for recognition

You may also see part of your role as helping to increase the credibility of aromatherapy and assist its integration with orthodox medical practices. In order to do so, you will need to consider the following:

- Foster a professional working relationship with all practitioners.

- Be accurate and well informed about your therapy.

- Avoid making unclear and unfounded statements regarding aromatherapy.

- Take an active role in the activities of your aromatherapy association.

- Consider conducting your own research.

- Respect the expertise and authority of others.

WIDENING YOUR HORIZONS

Exploring new territories

Your aromatherapy career may open doors to other challenges and life experiences. Thus it is useful to retain an open mind and consider all openings that present themselves. With the aid of an action plan, you can constructively work towards creating the opportunities you seek. New pathways may include:

- writing
- media involvement
- management opportunities
- product line development
- educational activities
- travel.

Going back to the basics

Throughout this book, you have read about the importance of the golden keys to success:

- careful planning
- preparation
- drive
- commitment
- belief in yourself
- enthusiasm
- humour.

These keys are not unique to building a successful career in aromatherapy; they are applicable to any challenge or new opportunity. Take these positive steps to realising your dreams.

SUMMARY

Regular evaluation of your direction and achievements is a healthy part of personal and professional development. The next step is to move forward and embrace the future. This chapter encourages you to:

- assess objectively your progress and achievements
- refer back to your original aims, objectives and motives

- consider financial planning for the future

- combine pride with humility

- honour your professional commitments

- create an action plan for changes and new challenges

- apply the basic principles of success to new situations.

CASE STUDIES

Jane enjoys the fruits of her labours

After three years of successful practice and enormous experience, Jane has decided to take on a new role. Now engaged to be married, she has invested in buying a long lease on premises in a prominent location in order to establish a natural healthcare clinic. Jane plans to reduce her own clinic hours, employ a receptionist and rent out clinic rooms to existing practitioners. Her long-term goal is to be the owner of a successful natural healthcare clinic and to devote more time to her home life.

Theresa strikes the right balance

Reflecting on the three years since embarking upon her aromatherapy career, Theresa feels satisfied with her life. She is managing to fund her voluntary work through the income from her home-based clinic and has greater self-esteem and confidence in relating to others. As a result of her further studies, her treatments tend to be a combined approach rather than pure aromatherapy. A welcome consequence of her work is that her social circle has widened. This has helped her to 'fill in the gap' now that her children have left home.

Mark taps into a lucrative market

Looking back over the past three years, Mark acknowledges that all has not been easy. His drive to succeed and positive approach have helped him deal with isolation and the difficulties of creating a respected niche for himself. His tenacity has ensured that he is now able truly to benefit from this commitment. He has expanded his clinic space at the leisure centre in order to train others in sports aromatherapy. He has been interviewed for television and radio and has attracted a number of world class athletes as his regular clients. His opportunities to lecture abroad continue.

THINKING IT THROUGH

1. What impact has the decision to become an aromatherapist had upon your life as a whole?

2. What is on your list of desires?

3. What is written on your current action plan?

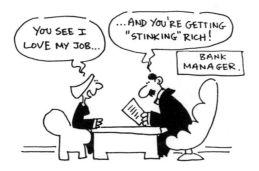

Glossary

Absorption. The process whereby essential oil components enter the body. Their chemical composition favours penetration of the skin and the mucous membranes of the respiratory tract.

Aesthetic. In aromatherapy terms, this is related to the use of essential oils for their effects in skin and beauty care.

Aroma chologist. An aroma chologist works with the effects of fragrance on the mind. This includes essential oils in addition to other fragrance products that may be synthetic in origin.

Aromatherapist. Someone who has undertaken and successfully completed training in the art and science of aromatherapy.

Aromatherapy. A therapy that utilises the therapeutic properties of essential oils in a variety of applications such as massage.

Aromatherapy associations. Independent bodies set up to support professional aromatherapists, monitor the therapy, develop training standards and promote aromatherapy to the general public. They usually give membership to aromatherapists who have completed approved levels of training and represent colleges who adhere to their standards and guidelines.

Aromatologist. An aromatologist uses essential oils for their therapeutic properties in clinical applications that may or may not include aromatherapy massage.

Base oil. Also termed a **fixed** or **carrier** oil, these are non-volatile vegetable oils that are used for their properties and qualities in skin care and their suitability for diluting essential oils for aromatherapy massage. Examples include sweet almond and macadamia nut oils.

Bioactivity. Essential oils are bioactive substances as they have a range of effects upon the mind and tissues of the body and demonstrate antimicrobial properties.

Blending. The process by which essential oils are combined to create a blend that is pleasing to smell and therapeutic in activity.

Concentrated. Essential oils are concentrated substances requiring substantial amounts of plant material to be distilled for their extraction. They are thus used sparingly and usually in **dilution**.

Contraindications. There are times when aromatherapy or particular essential oils are not suitable for use with individual clients. These are ascertained through detailed consultation with the client regarding their general health and lifestyle.

Diffuser. As essential oils are volatile, they are readily used for fragrancing or airborne dispersion. There are several types of diffuser on the market that aid airborne dispersion. These range from simple heat-producing diffusers to more complex microdiffusers that mist the essential oil without heat.

Dilution. The concentration of essential oils is such that they are rarely used neat in aromatherapeutic applications. They are more often diluted in a suitable medium such as **base oil** for application to the skin. The degree of dilution is dependent upon the type of application and the individual client.

Dispersing agent. As essential oils are poorly soluble in water, dispersing agents are often used to incorporate them into water-based products and applications.

Distillation. The process by which essential oils are extracted from plants. The basic principles are that when heated together with water or steam, aromatic plants give off their volatile components that are later recaptured by recondensation.

Essence. A term that may have two meanings in aromatherapy. Firstly, it may refer to the volatile components within the plant before extraction by distillation. Secondly, it may refer to the citrus essences obtained by expression from the rind of citrus fruits.

Essential oil. A collection of the volatile principles of plants from the same botanical origin by the process of **distillation**. A pure essential oil is one that has not been tampered with, diluted or adjusted in any way following distillation.

Hydrolat. Also termed **hydrosol** or **floral water**, this is a product of the same **distillation** process that yields essential oils. The recondensed water at the end of the process contains soluble and aromatic compounds that impart their fragrance and therapeutic properties.

Integral dropper insert. An orifice reducer present in each bottle of essential oil that allows the oil to be dispensed in drops. It also serves as a safety feature to prevent accidental ingestion.

Irritation. Essential oils are concentrated substances that can irritate the skin and mucous membranes if used inappropriately. Certain essential oils are more irritant than others. This is largely due to their chemical composition.

Latin name. Also termed the **botanical** or **binomial** name, this is the correct botanic nomenclature denoting the genus and species of a plant. It avoids the ambiguity and confusion that results when the common names of plants are used.

Massage. A method of manipulation of the soft tissues of the body, using a number of techniques such as frictions, kneading and stroking. There are many different massage styles taught around the world. Massage is often used in combination with aromatherapy to apply the chosen essential oil blend.

Notes. Taken from the realm of perfumery, the odour notes classification of fragrance can be applied to essential oils. Each essential oil has its own **top**, **middle** and **base** notes dependent upon the aroma and volatility of its various components. This is a useful tool for the aromatherapist to aid essential oil **blending**.

Oxidation. A chemical reaction and one of the processes that contribute to the degradation of an essential oil or base oil. Protection from exposure to air will slow the oxidation process.

Sense of smell. Also termed **olfaction**, the sense of smell is particularly relevant in the practice of aromatherapy. It is intimately connected with the conscious and subconscious mind, influencing memory, emotions, behaviour and hormonal activity.

Sensitisation. A process by which a person becomes allergic to a given substance. This can happen in aromatherapy and most commonly leads to skin reactions such as dermatitis. Sensitisation can develop over a period of time with repeated exposure to the potential allergen.

Synergy. In aromatherapy, this relates to the concept that an essential oil is the combined sum of its individual components, all of which contribute to its overall aroma and therapeutic effect. This concept is taken further when blending several essential oils together; it is thought that a greater synergetic effect is created when the oils are in combination than when used on their own.

Volatility. Essential oils are volatile substances. Volatility relates to the rate at which an essential oil evaporates.

Further Reading

There is an abundance of aromatherapy texts available for the therapist and lay person alike. Your aromatherapy college will provide you with a recommended reading list. You will form your own opinion as to the books you find most helpful. This section is concerned with giving you a starting point for further reading into other topics raised in the course of this book that concern the wider aspects of the therapy.

Practical Research – a Guide for Therapists, French, S. (Skills for Practice Series. Butterworth Heinmann Ltd, 1993).

Planning a Research Project: a Guide for Practitioners and Trainees in the Helping Professions, Herbert, M. (Cassell Educational Ltd, 1990).

Healthy Business, the Natural Practitioner's Guide to Success, Harland, M. and Finn, G. (Hyden House Ltd, 1990).

Teaching Adults, Rogers, A. (Open University Press, 1994).

Experiential Research: a New Paradigm, Heron, J. (Human Potential Research Project, University of Surrey, 1981).

Learning to Counsel. How to develop the skills to work effectively with others, Sutton, J. and Stewart, W. (How To Books, 1997).

Complementary Medicine Today: Practitioners and Patients, Sharma, U. (Routledge, 1991).

The Greening of Medicine, Pietrioni, P. C. (Gollancz, 1990).

Can I See the Records? Clinical notes–disclosure and patient access, Hoyte, P. (Medical Defence Union Ltd, 1996).

Problems in General Practice – Confidentiality, Schütte, P. (Medical Defence Union Ltd, 1997).

Useful Addresses and Resource Guide

AROMATHERAPY ASSOCIATIONS AND ORGANISATIONS IN THE UK

Aromatherapy Organisations Council (AOC), PO Box 19834, London SE25 6WF. Tel: (0208) 251 7912. Internet: www.aromatherapy-uk.org The UK governing body for aromatherapy. Implemented standards for the profession in 1994. Members include professional aromatherapy associations and colleges.

Aromatherapy Trade Council (ATC), PO Box 387, Ipswich, IP2 9AN. Tel & fax: (01473) 603630. Internet: www.a-t-c.org.uk The UK body for the aromatherapy essential oil trade. Members include essential oil suppliers who comply with the council's code of practice regarding marketing, product labelling, bottling and packaging.

International Society of Professional Aromatherapists (ISPA), ISPA House, 82 Ashby Road, Hinckley, Leicestershire LEIO 1SN. Tel: (01455) 637 987. Fax: (01455) 890 956.

Register of Qualified Aromatherapists (RQA), PO Box 3431, Danbury, Chelmsford, Essex CM3 4UA Tel: (01245) 227957.

The International Federation of Aromatherapists (IFA), Stamford House, 182 Chiswick High Road, Chiswick, London W4 1PP. Tel: (0208) 742 2605. Fax: (0208) 742 2606.
Internet: www.int-fed-aromatherapy.co.uk

The Institute of Aromatic Therapists, 4 Woodland Road, Hinckley, Leicestershire LE1O 1JG.

Guild of Complementary Practitioners (GCP), Liddell House, Liddell Close, Finchampstead, Berkshire RG40 4NS. Tel: (0118) 973 5757. Fax: (0118) 973 5767. Internet: www.gcpnet.com

AROMATHERAPY ASSOCIATIONS AND ORGANISATIONS OUTSIDE THE UK

Canadian Federation of Aromatherapists, 868 Markharn Road, Suite 109, Scarborough, Ontario M1H 2Y2, Canada. Tel: (416) 439 1951. Fax: (416) 439 4984.

Japan Aromatherapy Association, 1-5-1-302 Fujimi, Chiyoda-ku, Tokyo 102, Japan. Tel: (03) 3230 2922. Fax: (03) 3230 3008.

New Zealand Register of Holistic Aromatherapists, PO Box 18399, Glen Innes, Auckland 6, New Zealand.

Association of Aromatherapists Southern Africa, PO Box 23924, Claremont, Cape Town 7735 Republic of South Africa. Tel: (21) 5317314. E-mail: aoas@aglobal.co.za.

National Association for Holistic Aromatherapy (NAHA), 2000 2nd Avenue, Suite 206, Seattle, WA 98121 USA. Tel: (206) 256 0741 or 888-ASK-NAHA. Fax: (206) 770 5915. E-mail: info@naha.org Internet: www.naha.org

Aromatherapy Research Group, 15 Bayview Road Canada Bay, New South Wales 2046, Australia. Tel: (02) 97 44 6642. E-mail: ejbowles@speednet.com.au

Forum Essenzia, Mäuselweg 29, 81375 München, Germany. The German Aromatherapy Association.

UK ORGANISATIONS RELATING TO ALTERNATIVE AND COMPLEMENTARY MEDICINE

Institute for Complementary Medicine (ICM), PO Box 194, London SE16 7QZ. Tel: (0207) 237 5165. Internet: www.icmedicine.co.uk An independent charity since 1982, the ICM provides information on complementary medicine to the general public. Set up the British Register of Complementary Practitioners in 1989. This is open to qualified, insured practitioners who abide by the institute's code of conduct and practice.

British Complementary Medicine Association (BCMA), Kensington House, 33 Imperial Square, Cheltenham, Gloucestershire GL50 1QZ. Tel: (01242) 251 9911. Set up in 1990, it has a similar role to the ICM. The BCMA provides a consultative body for complementary medicine and has its own code of conduct and practice and register of members.

Council for Complementary and Alternative Medicine (CCAM), 63 Jeddow Road, London W12 98Q. Tel: (0208) 735 0632. Provides a forum for communication and co-operation between professional bodies, particularly in relation to education, ethics and discipline. Main therapies currently represented by CCAM are homeopathy, acupuncture, herbalism and osteopathy.

Research Council for Complementary Medicine (RCCM), 505 Riverbank House, 1 Putney Bridge Approach, London SW6 3JD. E-mail: info@rccm.org.uk Internet: www.rccm.org.uk Encourages and sponsors research into complementary medicine. Provides help with literature searches and guidance regarding research methodology.

Royal College of Nursing, Complementary Therapies Special Interest Group, 20 Cavendish Square, London W1M 0DB.

The British Holistic Medical Association (BHMA), Trust House, Royal Shrewsbury Hospital South, Shrewsbury SY3 8XF. Organisation for professionals interested in holistic medicine.

SCIENTIFIC RESEARCH

The Aromatherapy Database – research into the psychophysiological properties of essential oils and their components, Essential Oil Resource Consultants, 83840 La Martre, Provence, France. Tel/fax: (33) 494 84 29 93. E-mail: essentialorc@cs.com Published in English, this is a unique reference source updated annually from scientific journals worldwide.

The Aromatherapy Organisations Council (AOC), PO Box 19834, London SE25 6WF. Tel: (0208) 251 7912. Publishes guidelines for aromatherapists wishing to undertake research.

UK AROMATHERAPY JOURNALS

The International Journal of Aromatherapy, Journals Marketing Dept, Harcourt Publishers Ltd, Bewlay House, 32 Jamestown Road, London NW1 7BY. E-Mail: journals@harcourt.com Internet: www.harcourt-international.com

The Aromatherapist, SPA Ltd, Essentia House, Upper Bond Street, Hinckley, Leicestershire LE1O 1RS. Tel: (01455) 615466. Fax: (01455) 615054.

Aromatherapy Times, Stamford House, 182 Chiswick High Road, Chiswick, London W4 1PP. Tel: (0208) 742 2605. Fax: (0208) 742 2606.

Aromatheraphy World, ISPA House, 82 Ashby Road, Hinckley, Leicestershire, LE10 1SN. Tel: (01455) 637987. Fax: (01455) 890956.

AROMATHERAPY JOURNALS PUBLISHED OUTSIDE THE UK

Aroma News, Chausée Maïer Habils, 16-1430 Bierghes (Rebecq), Belgium. Tel: (32) 2 395 6053. Bimonthly newsletter of Natural Aromatherapy Research and Development (NARD), published in English, French or Japanese.

NAHA Aromatherapy Journal (formerly *Scensitivity*), 2000 2nd Avenue, Suite 206, Seattle WA 98121, USA. Tel: (206) 256 0741. Fax: (206) 770 5915. E-mail: info@naha.org

Fragrance Journal, 1F Seibunkan Building, 1-5-9 Idabashi, Chiyoda-ku, Tokyo 102-0072, Japan. Tel: (03) 3264 0125. Fax: (03) 3264 0148. Internet: www.nisiq.net/~fragra-j Publishers of the journal *Aromatopia* (in Japanese).

Aromatherapy Today, PO Box 211, Kellyville, New South Wales 2115, Australia. Tel: (02) 9894 9933. Fax: (02) 9894 0199. E-Mail: sales@aromatherapytoday.com

NATURAL HEALTH JOURNALS

Alternatives in Health, Freepost ANG 0805, Shenley, Radlett, Herts, WD7 9BR UK. Tel: 01923 856222

Positive Health, 51 Queen Square, Bristol BS1 4LH Tel: (0117) 983 8851. Fax: (0117) 908 0097. Internet: http://www.positive health.com.

Massage and Health Review, Lower Ground Floor, York Street Chambers, 68/72 York Street, London W1H 1DF. Published by the Massage Therapy Institute of Great Britain in conjunction with the Institute of Health Sciences.

Complementary Therapies in Medicine, Journals Marketing Dept, Harcourt Publishers Ltd, Bewlay House, 32 Jamestown Road, London NW1 7BY. E-Mail: journals@harcourt.com Internet: www.harcourt-international.com

Herbalgram, The Journal of the American Botanical Council and the Herb Research Foundation, PO Box 144345, Austin, Texas 78714-4345. Tel: (512) 926 4900. Fax: (512) 926 2345. E-Mail: custserv@herbalgram.org Internet: www.herbalgram.org

INSURANCE BROKERS

H&L Balen & Company, Specialist Insurance Brokers for Complementary Therapists and Organisations, 33 Graham Road,

Great Malvern, Worcs WR14 2HU. Tel: (01684) 893006. Fax: (01684) 893416.

LOANS, BUSINESS ASSOCIATIONS AND FINANCIAL ADVISERS

Career Development Loans. Information pack available from: The Department for Education and Employment, Career Development Loans, FREEPOST, Newcastle upon Tyne X NE85 1BR. CDLs available from Barclays, The Co-operative, Clydesdale and Royal Bank of Scotland.

The Small Business Bureau, Curzon House, Church Road, Windlesham, Surrey GU20 6BH. Tel: (01276) 452010. Fax: (01276 451602). E-mail: SBB@compuserve.com Internet: http://www.smallbusinessbureau.org.uk

Business Link. Business Link Signpost Line: (0345) 567 765. Set up by the Department of Trade and Industry. Provides advice on business and access to Independent Personal Business Advisers in your locality.

OTHERS

Local Government Management Board, Publications Department, Layden House, 76–86 Turnmill Street, London EC1M 5QU. Fax: (0207) 296 6523. Provides copies (not free) of the National Occupational Standards for Aromatherapy (ref. WS0129).

Small Firms Publications – the Department of Trade and Industry produces a range of free publications. List of publications available from: DTI, SME Policy Directorate, St Mary's House, c/o Moorfoot, Sheffield S1 4PQ.

WHICH? publications – tax-saving guides available from: Which?, Dept WOL97, FREEPOST, Herts X, SG14 1YB. E-mail: WHICH @WHICH.NET Internet: www.which.net/index.html

Stationery Office Publications Centre, Stationery Office Books, PO Box 276, London SW8 5DT. Internet:www.open.gov.uk/dpr/dprhome.htm. Provides copies of Acts such as the Data Protection Act.

Performing Rights Society, 29–33 Berners Street, London W1P 4AA. Tel: (0207) 580 5544. Fax: (0207) 306 4050. Internet: http://prs.co.uk

ACTPLAN. The first comprehensive private medical scheme for members of the public wishing to have cover for alternative and complementary therapies, including aromatherapy. IGI Insurance Company Ltd, FREEPOST (NG6660), Nottingham NG1 1BR. Helpline: (0800) 393033.

The Herb Society, 77 Great Peter Street, London SW1 2EZ. Produces a list of herbal suppliers and herb gardens. Also produces a quarterly magazine.

The Medical Defence Union, 3 Devonshire Place, London W1N 2EA. Tel: (0207) 486 6181. Publish booklets concerning record keeping and confidentiality.

Index

BECOMING A COMPLEMENTARY THERAPIST
How to start a career in the new caring professions

Linda Wilson

Aromatherapy, massage, reflexology, crystal healing, hypnotherapy and yoga are just a few of the therapies explored in this indispensable book. It shows you what training is required, helps you assess your suitability for different fields, and includes expert advice on setting up and running your own practice. 'Well-researched, well-written and informative . . . useful for thinking about your future career prospects.' *Newscheck*. Linda Wilson has her own practice and is a member of the International Federation of Aromatherapists. She is also trained in Reiki, Shen Tao acupressure and macrobiotics.

144pp. illus. 1 85703 628 X 2nd edition

WORKING AS A NURSE
How to make your career in a fulfilling profession

Esther Bartlett and Marion Field

Explore the variety of work available in this changing profession and discover the options for gaining qualifications through this user-friendly book. It covers work in hospitals, the community, in industry and abroad, as well as other nursing-related careers. Marion Field teams her extensive writing credentials with Esther Bartlett's substantial NHS nursing and research experience.

144pp. illus. 1 85703 443 0.

WORKING IN THE VOLUNTARY SECTOR
How to find rewarding work with charities and voluntary organisations

Craig Brown

Whatever your age or skills, whether you want to work full time, part time, or just a few hours a week, this invaluable guide tells you what you need to know. 'Packed with accessible information and written from the author's years of experience and recruitment in the voluntary sector . . . suitable for Year 11 upwards, and adults considering this kind of work' *Newscheck*. '. . . describes the benefits of working for a charity and the different types of work available – be it paid or unpaid in the UK or overseas.' *Streetwyse.*

136pp. illus. 1 85703 367 1

WORKING FOR THE ENVIRONMENT
How to make a career of caring for the world we live in

Barbara Buffton

'[A] detailed and impartial overview of all types of work in the UK environmental/countryside sector. [It] is the most comprehensive account I have come across and covers the Who, What, Where, When, How and Why of the most important career in the world.' *Niall Carson, Countryside Jobs Service.* 'Covers courses, jobs and careers available throughout the environmental industry.' *The Job Hunter's Guide.*

144pp. illus. 1 85703 366 3.